A Practical Guide to Beating Cancer

Combining Natural Therapies with Conventional Care for Optimal Healing

Tru Wayne, Naturopath

Tru Wayne

Copyright © 2024 by Tru Wayne. All rights reserved.

The contents of this book may not be reproduced, duplicated, or transmitted without direct written permission from the author.

Under no circumstances will any legal responsibility or blame be held against the publisher for any reparation, damages, or monetary loss due to the information herein, either directly or indirectly.

Legal Notice:

This book is copyright-protected. This is only for personal use. You cannot amend, distribute, sell, use, quote, or paraphrase any part of the content within this book without the consent of the author.

Disclaimer Notice:

Please note the information contained within this document is for educational purposes only. Every attempt has been made to provide accurate, up-to-date, and reliable complete information. No warranties of any kind are expressed or implied. Readers acknowledge that the author is not engaging in the rendering of legal, financial, medical, or professional advice. The content of this book has been derived from various sources. Please consult a licensed professional before attempting any techniques outlined in this book.

By reading this document, the reader agrees that under no circumstances is the author responsible for any losses, direct or indirect, which are incurred as a result of the use of the information contained within this document, including, but not limited to, —errors, omissions, or inaccuracies.

Contents

Preface   1

Introduction   4

1. Understanding Cancer   7
   What Is Cancer
   How Does Cancer Develop
   Differences between Normal Cells and Cancer Cells
   Stages of cancer development
   Common Causes and Risk Factors
   Debunking Common Myths about Cancer
   The Importance of Early Detection
   Taking Control through Understanding

2. Diagnosing Cancer   15
   Factors That Affect Diagnosis
   Common Early Symptoms
   Common diagnostic methods:

3. Conventional Cancer Treatments   21

4. Standard Treatment of Common Cancers   31

5. Conventional Treatments Need Complementary Help Why?   64

How Natural Therapies can help

Common anti-cancer products in natural therapies

6. Navigating Potential Risks - Avoiding Harmful Interactions — 98

    Practical Guidance for Safety

    Common Unwanted Interactions listed by natural products

7. Combined Therapies for Common cancers — 112

    Breast Cancer:

    Lung Cancer

    Liver Cancer

    Colon or Colorectal Cancer

    Pancreatic Cancer

    Gastric or Stomach Cancer

    Prostate Cancer

    Brain cancer

    Skin Cancer (Melanoma)

    How these natural products are prepared and used.

8. Nutrition and Diet: Fueling Your Fight — 154

    Foods to Avoid

    Foods to Support Cancer Treatment

    Meal time and meal size

    Benefits of the of healthy diet for cancer treatment

    Testimonials from Cancer Patients

    Practical Meal Plans and Tips for Maintaining a Balanced Diet

    Meal Planning:

    Weekly Meal Plan Example

9. Mind and Body Healing: Finding Strength from Within — 164

    Believing, Hoping, and Staying Confident

Cultivating Hope, Confidence, and Calm
   Relaxation and Physical Activities to Support Healing
   Physical Activity for Well-being
   Building a Daily Practice

10. Step-by-Step Guide to combining natural and standard   175
    therapies
       Consultation Tips

Conclusion   186

Sources of Information: 190

Appendix 1   193
   Aloe arborescens
   Bitter Melon
   Black Cumin
   Blueberries
   Flaxseeds
   Fucoidan
   Garlic

Appendix 2   232
   Ginger
   Honey
   Mistletoe
   Papaya leaves and seeds
   Perilla leaves and seed oil
   Probiotics and Fermented Foods
   Turmeric
   Virgin Coconut Oil

Preface

After retiring in 2010, I looked for opportunities to participate in volunteer work. However, after more than a year, I couldn't find any suitable opportunities. Witnessing and hearing about so many people suffering from chronic illnesses—conditions that modern medicine not only failed to cure but could even worsen—I was heartbroken. It was even more painful to hear about acquaintances near and far who suffered from cancer, undergoing treatments, only to pass away shortly after. So, I enrolled in a college of natural therapies program to gain the knowledge needed to help me avoid chronic illnesses and help those facing such situations.

After graduating, I volunteered as a naturopath at Antara Free Natural Health Clinic, mainly for low income people, in Auckland. While caring for patients and conducting extensive research into natural therapies for chronic illnesses, I focused particularly on cancer, reading almost all the research available on natural therapies for the disease. I was delighted to learn that thousands of studies had explored herbs, plants, fruits, and natural products used to treat cancer. Together with healthy eating and physical activity, many people had successfully treated cancer using natural therapies.

I also researched and listened to the experiences shared by cancer survivors identifying the core principles common to their success. I worked hard to share these findings online and applied these therapies for many cancer patients who had either completed or were undergoing conventional treatments. The results were very positive. All patients avoided side effects such as hair loss, fatigue, weakness, nausea, and loss of appetite, while the tumors gradually disappeared.

The younger sister of a friend of mine in the United States suffered from metastatic pancreatic cancer. Due to metastases from the pancreatic cancer, her right lung had six tumors, and her left lung had three tumors. After three months of chemotherapy combined with natural therapies along the line of this guide, her right lung had only five tumors remaining, and the blood vessels supplying these tumors had dried up. Her left lung was down to just one tumor, giving much hope for completely treating this dangerous cancer.

Thanh, the wife of another friend of mine, was diagnosed with colon cancer. She combined natural therapies with surgery. She is now cancer-free and healthy.

Stories like these demonstrate that integrating natural and conventional medical treatments can bring hope for curing cancer.

Without the support of natural therapies, conventional treatments often fail to deliver the desired outcomes, particularly in advanced stages (stages III and IV) or metastatic cases. Several people I know personally passed away shortly after undergoing chemotherapy and radiation. Moreover, while undergoing conventional treatment, they lived in misery due to the side effects of these therapies.

Conventional cancer treatments are most effective when cancer is detected early. However, in cases where cancer is diagnosed late, these treatments often fail to save lives and cause patients to suffer from harsh side effects. Many studies, clinical evidence, and my experience indicate that natural therapies can enhance the effectiveness of conventional treatments while also reducing their side effects.

Testimonies from cancer survivors also highlight the significant role of natural therapies, including belief and confidence in the body's healing ability, healthy eating, and physical activity, in the journey to overcoming cancer.

However, there is no clear guide for cancer patients and their families on how to integrate these approaches safely and effectively.

That's why I've written this practical guide. My hope is that it will provide clarity, support, and hope to those on the challenging journey of fighting cancer, as well as to their loved ones. This book aims to empower you with knowledge, resources and step-by-step guide so you can participate actively in your treatment plan, advocate for integrative approaches with your healthcare team, and, most importantly, find healing and peace.

Introduction

Any of us diagnosed with cancer, along with our families, face a challenging journey. We can take control of this journey by gaining the necessary knowledge and taking a proactive approach. We need to explore every available option and understand each step in the process. This proactive approach not only gives us a sense of control but also helps us feel more prepared for what lies ahead, and it can make all the difference.

This book *A Practical Guide to Beating Cancer * is designed to be your companion through this challenging journey. It has ten chapters, each focusing on different aspects of cancer care—from understanding the nature of cancer and exploring conventional treatments to integrating natural therapies and making informed decisions for your health and for supporting your loved ones.

This book provides a balanced, research-backed approach to combining conventional cancer treatments with natural therapies. Many cancer patients and their families are not aware of the significant benefits that natural approaches can offer when integrated thoughtfully into standard medical care. Combining these two worlds can enhance treatment effectiveness, minimize side effects, and improve your or your loved ones' quality of life.

Throughout this book, you will learn about cancer, how it develops, and the role both conventional and natural treatments can play and why they should be combined holistically. You will gain insight into the different types of traditional therapies available, as well as natural, plant-based therapies that have shown promise in supporting treatment and reducing side effects. This guide will help you understand how to navigate the complexities of cancer care, make informed decisions, and actively participate in your treatment plan or support your loved one's journey back to normal health.

The first four chapters will focus on how cancer develops, how it is diagnosed, how conventional therapies treat cancer in general and what treatments are commonly used for specific cancers. Why conventional need complementary help from natural therapies and how natural therapies can help, including potential risks of unwanted interactions will be presented in chapters 5 -6. Recommended combined therapies for common cancers will be presented in chapter 7, which may be helpful to be read first if you are undergoing or have ended standard treatment. The role of healthy diet and mind body activities will be in chapters 8 and 9. A step-by-step guide of the whole journey is in chapter 10,

I aim to provide practical, easy-to-understand information to help you regain control in discussing the treatment plan with your oncologist. You deserve to feel empowered and confident as you progress to optimum healing. Whether you are just beginning your treatment or looking for ways to improve your or your loved one's current approach, this book is here to give you clarity, comfort, and actionable steps that can make a difference.

With this guide, you will be confident to discuss with your oncologist about incorporating natural therapies into the treatment plan instead of just asking for their opinion or permission.

Remember, this journey is not one you or your loved one must take alone. Together with your healthcare team, you can explore the options, make informed choices, and work toward the best possible outcome that emphasizes healing, quality of life, and hope.

If you are caring for your loved ones with cancer or are interested in looking to avoid cancer, the natural anticancer products, healthy diet and lifestyle habits presented in chapters 5, 8 and 9 can not only support cancer treatment but also help prevent cancer from developing in the first place.

If you or your loved ones have undergone conventional treatment and are struggling with its adverse effects, this book will help you recover more effectively and without fear of recurrence.

****

Chapter 1

Understanding Cancer

U nderstanding the nature of cancer is the first step toward winning the battle. Gain knowledge, reduce fear, and prepare for the fight.

Cancer is a word that evokes fear, uncertainty, and confusion for many of us. But understanding what cancer is, how it develops, and why it behaves the way it does can help reduce some of that fear and give us a sense of empowerment. Knowledge is the first step toward taking control of your treatment and being an active participant in your healing journey.

What Is Cancer?

Cancer is a disease characterized by the uncontrolled growth and spread of abnormal cells in the body. Normally, our cells grow, divide, and die in a regulated way. However, when the body loses control over this process, cells begin to grow uncontrollably, forming a mass called a tumor. Not all tumors are cancerous—benign tumors do not spread to other parts of the body, while malignant tumors can invade nearby tissues and spread to distant areas.

Cancer can develop in nearly any part of the body, and there are more than 100 types of cancer, each named for the organ or cell type in which it originates. Some of the most common cancers include breast, lung, prostate, and colorectal cancers, but many others affect different tissues and organs.

How Does Cancer Develop?

Cancer begins when a cell's DNA becomes damaged or mutated. DNA is the genetic blueprint that controls how our cells function. Mutations can be caused by a variety of factors, such as exposure to certain chemicals, radiation, lifestyle choices like smoking, or even inherited genetic predispositions. When DNA is damaged, and the body's repair mechanisms fail, cells may begin to grow and divide uncontrollably.

Stem Cells in the Development of Cancer

Stem cells play a crucial role in the development of cancer. These are cells that have the potential to differentiate into various cell types and the ability to self-renew. In the context of cancer, cancer stem cells are believed to be responsible for initiating and sustaining tumor growth. These cancer stem cells are more resistant to conventional treatments like chemotherapy and radiation, which target rapidly dividing cells but may not effectively eliminate the cancer stem cells. As a result, these stem cells can survive and lead to recurrence or metastasis, making cancer harder to treat in the long term.

Eliminating cancer stem cells (CSCs) is considered critical in cancer treatment due to their unique ability to initiate, sustain, and regenerate tumors, as well as their resistance to many conventional therapies. Unlike most cancer cells that divide rapidly, CSCs are slow-cycling, making them less vulnerable to standard chemotherapy and radiation treatments, which primarily target fast-dividing cells. This resistance allows CSCs to survive treatment, potentially leading to recurrence and metastasis as they can repopulate the tumor even after the majority of other cancer cells are eliminated.

Current therapies struggle to completely eradicate CSCs because these cells often possess robust DNA repair mechanisms, enabling them to survive traditional treatments and even adapt to evade them.

What Is Metastasis?

Metastasis is the process by which cancer spreads from the original site to other parts of the body. Cancer cells can break away from the primary tumor and travel through the bloodstream or the lymphatic system to form new tumors in other organs. This spread makes cancer more difficult to treat and is often responsible for the most severe complications. Unlike normal cells, cancer cells can invade nearby tissues and adapt to new environments, allowing them to establish secondary tumors. Common sites for metastasis include the bones, liver, lungs, and brain.

Differences between Normal Cells and Cancer Cells

Growth: Normal cells grow, divide, and die in a regulated manner. Cancer cells, on the other hand, grow uncontrollably and do not respond to the signals that regulate normal cell division. This uncontrolled growth leads to tumor formation.

Behavior: Normal cells have specific functions within the body and stop dividing once their role is complete. Cancer cells lose these specialized functions and continue dividing indefinitely. They can also evade the body's natural cell death mechanisms, allowing them to survive longer than normal cells.

Structure: Cancer cells often have an abnormal structure compared to normal cells. Their size and shape may vary significantly, and their nuclei (the control centers of the cells) are typically larger and darker due to excess genetic material.

Interaction with the Body: Normal cells communicate with each other to maintain balance within tissues. Cancer cells lose this ability and can invade surrounding tissues. They can also manipulate the body's blood supply, forming new blood vessels (a process called angiogenesis) to provide themselves with nutrients and oxygen, aiding in their growth and spread.

Drug Resistance: Cancer cells can develop resistance to drugs, making treatment more challenging over time. This drug resistance can occur due to several mechanisms, such as genetic mutations that alter drug targets, increased ability to pump drugs out of cells, or the activation of alternative signaling pathways to bypass the effects of treatment. These adaptations allow cancer cells to survive even in the presence of chemotherapy, necessitating the use of combination therapies or newer targeted treatments to overcome resistance.

Functionality: Normal cells perform specific, specialized functions within the body, such as producing hormones or supporting immune responses. Cancer cells, however, often lose these specialized functions, becoming less efficient and more focused on growth and division rather than fulfilling their original roles.

Genetic Stability: Normal cells maintain genetic stability with fewer mutations over time. Cancer cells, in contrast, exhibit high genetic instability and accumulate numerous mutations, which contribute to their uncontrolled growth and ability to evade normal regulatory mechanisms.

Mutations: Mutations in normal cells are typically repaired by the body's natural repair mechanisms, preventing abnormal growth. Cancer cells, however, often acquire multiple mutations that allow them to grow uncontrollably. These mutations may affect genes that regulate cell division, DNA repair, or apoptosis (programmed cell death).

Lifespan: Normal cells have a limited lifespan and will undergo apoptosis once they are damaged or old. Cancer cells, however, develop mechanisms to evade apoptosis, effectively becoming 'immortal.' This allows them to continue dividing indefinitely, contributing to tumor growth.

Energy Production and Metabolism: Normal cells primarily generate energy through a process called aerobic respiration, using oxygen to produce ATP, the energy currency of cells efficiently. Cancer cells, however, rely heavily on glycolysis, even in the presence of oxygen, a phenomenon known as the Warburg effect. This metabolic shift allows cancer cells to rapidly produce energy and build the molecules needed for quick growth but is far less efficient compared to normal cellular metabolism.

Response to the Immune System: The immune system usually recognizes and tolerates normal cells. When a normal cell becomes damaged or functions abnormally, the immune system often identifies and eliminates it. Cancer cells, however, develop ways to evade the immune system. They can create an environment that suppresses immune responses or disguise themselves to avoid detection. This ability to escape immune surveillance makes cancer more challenging to control.

Stages of cancer development:

The process of cancer development can be broken down into several stages:

1. Initiation: This is when a normal cell's DNA is damaged, creating a potential for cancerous growth.

2. Promotion: During this Stage, certain factors—such as lifestyle, diet, and exposure to toxins—encourage the mutated cells to grow and divide.

3. **Progression**: In this final Stage, the mutated cells grow rapidly, forming a tumor that can invade nearby tissues and spread to other parts of the body through the bloodstream or lymphatic system.

Common Causes and Risk Factors

Understanding the common causes and risk factors of cancer can help us take preventive steps where possible. Some risk factors are out of our control, such as genetics, while others are related to lifestyle choices and environmental exposures. Here are some of the most well-known risk factors for cancer:

Genetics: Certain gene mutations can be inherited, which may increase the risk of developing specific types of cancer. For example, BRCA1 and BRCA2 gene mutations are linked to an increased risk of breast and ovarian cancer.

Lifestyle Choices: Smoking, excessive alcohol consumption, poor diet, and lack of physical activity are all factors that can increase cancer risk.

Environmental Exposures: Exposure to harmful chemicals, radiation, or pollution can increase the likelihood of developing cancer. For example, asbestos exposure is linked to mesothelioma, a type of lung cancer.

Infections: Certain infections, such as human papillomavirus (HPV), hepatitis B and C, and Helicobacter pylori, are associated with increased cancer risk.

While some risk factors are unavoidable, many can be reduced by making healthy lifestyle choices. Quitting smoking, eating a balanced diet rich in fruits and vegetables, exercising regularly, and minimizing exposure to harmful substances are all ways to reduce your risk.

Debunking Common Myths about Cancer

Misinformation about cancer is widespread, and it can add to the anxiety that people feel when faced with a diagnosis. Let's take a moment to debunk a few common myths:

Myth 1: Cancer Is Always Fatal: Many types of cancer are treatable and even curable, especially when detected early. Advances in treatment have improved survival rates significantly.

Myth 2: Cancer Is Contagious: Cancer is not contagious and cannot be spread from person to person. It is a result of genetic mutations within the body.

The Importance of Early Detection

Early detection of cancer greatly improves the chances of successful treatment. Paying attention to early symptoms of cancer is beneficial. Never downplay symptoms that may relate to cancer. Regular screenings, such as mammograms, colonoscopies, and skin checks, can help detect cancer at an early stage, often before symptoms appear. Knowing your family history and discussing it with your healthcare provider can also guide you in determining which screenings are most appropriate for you.

Taking Control through Understanding

Understanding cancer is the foundation of taking control of your health. It allows you to make informed decisions, understand treatment options, and advocate for yourself throughout your care. This chapter aimed to provide a basic understanding of what cancer is and how it develops, empowering you to face the journey ahead with greater confidence.

In the next chapter, we will explore the ways in which cancer is diagnosed, the importance of getting accurate information, and how to work effectively with your healthcare team to determine the best path forward. The more you know, the more prepared you will be to navigate the complexities of cancer care.

References:

1. National Cancer Institute. (2021). What Is Cancer?. Retrieved from https://www.cancer.gov/about-cancer/understanding/what-is-cancer

2. World Health Organization (WHO). (2022). Cancer: Key Facts. Retrieved from https://www.who.int/news-room/fact-sheets/detail/cancer

3. American Cancer Society. (2020). How Cancer Starts, Grows, and Spreads. Retrieved from https://www.cancer.org/cancer/cancer-basics/what-is-cancer.html

4. Hanahan, D., & Weinberg, R. A. (2011). Hallmarks of Cancer: The Next Generation. Cell, 144(5), 646-674.

5. Mayo Clinic. (2022). Cancer: Overview. Retrieved from https://www.mayoclinic.org/diseases-conditions/cancer/symptoms-causes/syc-20370588

Chapter 2

Diagnosing Cancer

Cancer diagnosis is a crucial step in determining the most effective treatment plan and improving the chances of recovery. An early and accurate diagnosis helps in understanding the Stage and progression of the disease, which in turn guides the best approach for treatment. In this chapter, we will explore the different methods of diagnosing cancer, factors that can affect the diagnosis, and how these processes differ based on the type of cancer.

Factors That Affect Diagnosis

Several factors can influence the process of diagnosing cancer. These include the patient's age, medical history, the type of symptoms they present, and the availability of advanced diagnostic tools. For example:

- *Medical History and Genetics*: A family history of certain cancers might prompt doctors to pursue more aggressive testing and earlier screening.

- *Symptoms*: Vague or nonspecific symptoms can delay diagnosis, whereas more pronounced symptoms can lead to faster identification of the disease.

- *Access to Medical Care*: The ability to access high-quality healthcare and advanced diagnostic tools can significantly impact how early and accurately cancer is diagnosed.

- *Type and Location of Cancer*: Cancers in certain organs, such as the brain or pancreas, are often harder to diagnose early due to the lack of clear symptoms or the location within the body.

Common Early Symptoms

Recognizing the early signs of cancer can lead to timely diagnosis and better outcomes. Common early symptoms vary depending on the type of cancer but may include:

Unexplained Weight Loss: Sudden and unexplained weight loss can be an early sign of cancers like pancreatic, stomach, or lung cancer.

Persistent Fatigue: Chronic fatigue that does not improve with rest can indicate cancers such as leukemia or colon cancer.

Lumps or Swelling: The presence of lumps, particularly in areas like the breast, neck, or armpits, should be evaluated promptly.

Changes in Skin: Skin changes, such as new moles, changes in existing moles, or non-healing sores, can be an early sign of skin cancer.

Persistent Cough or Difficulty Swallowing: Long-term cough or difficulty swallowing may indicate lung, throat, or esophageal cancer.

Questions to ask your doctor

When discussing your diagnosis with your doctor, consider asking the following questions to understand your condition better:

- What tests will be performed to confirm the diagnosis?

- How accurate are the diagnostic methods being used?

- What Stage is my cancer, and what does that mean for my treatment options?

- Should I get a second opinion?

- Are there any additional screenings or follow-up tests needed?

There are various methods that doctors use to diagnose cancer. The choice of method often depends on the type of cancer suspected and the patient's overall condition.

Common diagnostic methods:

Physical Examination: Doctors may start by looking for lumps or abnormal growths that could indicate a tumor.

Imaging Tests: Techniques such as X-rays, CT scans, MRIs, and ultrasounds are used to visualize abnormalities within the body.

Laboratory Tests: Blood and urine tests can provide important clues. Elevated levels of certain markers might indicate the presence of cancer.

Biopsy: A biopsy is one of the most definitive methods for diagnosing cancer. It involves taking a small sample of tissue from the suspicious area and examining it under a microscope to check for cancer cells.

Different Diagnosing Processes for Different Types of Cancer

The diagnostic process can vary significantly depending on the type of cancer. For example:

Blood Cancers: Blood cancers (Leukemia, Lymphoma) are diagnosed mainly through blood tests and bone marrow biopsies, which help detect abnormalities in blood cell counts.

Brain Cancer: Diagnosed using neurological exams, imaging tests such as MRIs or CT scans, and confirmed with a biopsy when possible.

Breast Cancer: Diagnosed primarily through mammograms and ultrasounds, followed by biopsies to confirm if a suspicious mass is cancerous.

Colorectal Cancer: Diagnosed through colonoscopy, which allows doctors to see inside the colon and take tissue samples for analysis

Gastric Cancer: Diagnosed through an endoscopy, where a camera is used to examine the stomach lining, along with biopsy samples taken for analysis

Liver Cancer: Typically diagnosed using imaging tests such as ultrasounds, CT scans, or MRIs, often followed by a biopsy to confirm the diagnosis.

Lung Cancer: Often diagnosed using imaging techniques such as chest X-rays and CT scans, with bronchoscopy or biopsy for confirmation.

Pancreatic Cancer: Diagnosed with imaging tests like CT scans or MRIs, and sometimes endoscopic ultrasound (EUS) combined with a biopsy.

Skin Cancer: Diagnosed through a physical examination of the skin, often followed by a biopsy of suspicious moles or lesions.

The Importance of an Accurate Diagnosis

Accurate diagnosis is essential for developing an effective treatment plan. Misdiagnosis or delayed diagnosis can lead to inappropriate treatment, which may reduce the chances of successful recovery. It is also important for the patient to seek a second opinion if they feel unsure about the results, as this can help confirm the diagnosis and ensure the right path forward.

Working with Your Healthcare Team

Diagnosing cancer can be overwhelming, but having a supportive healthcare team makes a big difference. Your healthcare team includes oncologists, radiologists, pathologists, and other specialists who work together to ensure you receive the best care. Feel free to ask questions, understand the tests being performed, and discuss all available options with your team.

In summary, diagnosing cancer is a complex process that depends on multiple factors, including the type of cancer, symptoms, and access to medical care. By understanding how cancer is diagnosed and the factors that affect the process, you can be better prepared to take an active role in your care. In the next chapter, we will discuss conventional cancer treatments and how they work, as well as the potential side effects and how they can be managed. Knowledge is power, and understanding your diagnosis is the first step toward making informed decisions about your treatment and care.

References:

1. National Cancer Institute. (2022). *Cancer Diagnosis Overview.*

Retrieved from https://www.cancer.gov/about-cancer/diagnosis-staging/diagnosis

2. American Cancer Society. (2021). *Cancer Screening and Diagnosis*. Retrieved from https://www.cancer.org/cancer/diagnosis-staging.html

3. World Health Organization (WHO). (2021). *Cancer Diagnosis and Staging Guidelines*. Retrieved from https://www.who.int/health-topics/cancer/diagnosis-and-treatment

4. Mayo Clinic. (2022). *Cancer Diagnosis: Procedures and Tests*. Retrieved from https://www.mayoclinic.org/diseases-conditions/cancer/diagnosis-treatment/drc-20370594

5. Johns Hopkins Medicine. (2020). *Cancer Diagnosis: Understanding Diagnostic Tests and Procedures*. Retrieved from https://www.hopkinsmedicine.org/cancer/diagnosis

Chapter 3

Conventional Cancer Treatments

Once cancer is diagnosed, the next step is to determine the most effective way to treat it. Conventional cancer treatments have been studied extensively in clinical trials and are widely used by healthcare professionals around the world. These treatments include surgery, radiation therapy, chemotherapy, targeted therapy, immunotherapy, and hormone therapy. Each treatment approach has its strengths, potential side effects, and suitability depending on the type and stage of cancer.

In this chapter, we will explore the different types of conventional cancer treatments, how they work, their advantages and disadvantages, and how they are often combined to provide the best possible outcomes for patients.

Surgery

Surgery is one of the most common treatments for cancer, especially when the tumor is localized. The primary goal of surgery is to remove the cancerous tumor physically and, if necessary, some surrounding tissue to ensure that no cancer cells remain. Surgery is often used in combination with other treatments, such as chemotherapy or radiation, to prevent recurrence.

Types of Surgery:

Depending on the type of cancer, there are various surgical techniques, including minimally invasive surgery (laparoscopic) and more extensive surgeries for larger tumors.

Surgery can be highly effective at removing localized tumors and can lead to a complete cure if the cancer has not spread.

However, surgery may not be an option if the cancer has metastasized or if the patient is not healthy enough to undergo an operation. Risks include infection, bleeding, and potential damage to surrounding organs.

Radiation Therapy

Radiation therapy uses high-energy rays to destroy cancer cells or inhibit their growth. It can be used alone or in combination with other treatments, like surgery or chemotherapy. It is often used for cancers that cannot be completely removed surgically or to reduce the size of tumors before surgery.

How it Works:

Radiation damages the DNA within cancer cells, making it impossible for them to grow and divide. This leads to the gradual death of cancer cells in the treated area.

It can effectively target specific areas of the body, minimizing the impact on healthy tissues.

However, radiation may have *side effects*, including fatigue, skin changes, and localized pain. Long-term risks include damage to nearby organs and tissues.

Chemotherapy

Chemotherapy involves the use of powerful drugs to kill cancer cells or stop them from growing. It is often used to treat cancers that have spread to multiple parts of the body and can be administered orally or intravenously.

How It Works: Chemotherapy drugs target rapidly dividing cells, which include both cancer cells and some healthy cells, such as those in the hair follicles and digestive tract. Chemotherapy drugs work through various mechanisms to effectively kill cancer cells or prevent them from growing. It is useful to know which mechanisms are used by chemotherapy drugs and which ones can have adverse interactions with natural products.

Oxidative Stress Inducers: Some chemotherapy drugs work by generating high levels of reactive oxygen species (ROS) within cancer cells, creating oxidative stress that damages cellular components such as DNA, proteins, and lipids. This overwhelming damage leads to the death of the cancer cells. Examples include anthracyclines like doxorubicin, which are known to induce oxidative stress as part of their mechanism of action.

Alkylating Agents:

These drugs work by damaging the DNA of cancer cells, which prevents them from replicating and eventually leads to cell death. Alkylating agents also induce oxidative stress, which increases cellular damage and contributes to cancer cell death. Alkylating agents can affect all phases of the cell cycle and are effective against a wide range of cancers.

Antimetabolites:

These drugs mimic the natural substances that cells need to build DNA and RNA. By replacing these natural substances, antimetabolites interfere with cancer cell division and growth. Common examples include *methotrexate and 5-fluorouracil*.

Topoisomerase Inhibitors:

Topoisomerases are enzymes that help maintain the structure of DNA during cell division. Topoisomerase inhibitors cause breaks in the DNA strands, ultimately preventing cancer cells from dividing and growing. Examples include *irinotecan and etoposide*.

Mitotic Inhibitors interfere with the microtubules involved in cell division, effectively stopping cancer cells from completing mitosis, which leads to cell death. *Paclitaxel and vincristine* are examples of mitotic inhibitors.

Platinum-based Compounds:

Drugs such as cisplatin and Carboplatin create cross-links within the DNA of cancer cells, preventing them from replicating and leading to cell death. Platinum-based compounds also promote the generation of reactive oxygen species (ROS), leading to oxidative damage that contributes to cancer cell death.

Advantages: Chemotherapy can be effective in treating cancers that have metastasized, and it can shrink tumors before surgery or radiation.

Disadvantages: Chemotherapy affects healthy cells as well, it can cause significant side effects such as nausea, vomiting, hair loss, and weakened immune function.

Targeted Therapy

Targeted Therapy is a newer approach that specifically targets cancer cells based on their unique characteristics. Unlike chemotherapy, which affects all rapidly dividing cells, targeted therapies aim to attack only cancer cells, thereby *minimizing damage to healthy tissues.* These drugs interfere with specific molecules that cancer cells need to grow and survive, such as proteins or genes that drive cancer progression. Targeted therapy drugs use the following various mechanisms:

Monoclonal Antibodies:

Monoclonal antibodies are laboratory-made molecules designed to bind to specific proteins on the surface of cancer cells. By attaching to these proteins, monoclonal antibodies can mark cancer cells for destruction by the immune system or block signals that stimulate their growth. Examples include *trastuzumab*, used for HER2-positive breast cancer, and *rituximab*, used for certain types of lymphoma.

Tyrosine Kinase Inhibitors (TKIs): Tyrosine kinases (TKIs) are enzymes that play a key role in cell signaling and growth. Blocking these enzymes helps stop the growth and spread of cancer cells. Examples include *imatinib*, which is used to treat chronic myeloid leukemia (CML), and *erlotinib*, which is used for non-small cell lung cancer.

PARP Inhibitors: These drugs inhibit poly (ADP-ribose) polymerase (PARP), an enzyme involved in DNA repair.

PARP inhibitors block the repair of single-strand DNA breaks. In cancer cells that already have deficiencies in other DNA repair mechanisms (e.g., BRCA mutations), this leads to the accumulation of DNA damage and cell death. *Examples*: *Olaparib, Rucaparib, Niraparib*

Anti-Angiogenesis Drugs: These drugs inhibit the formation of new blood vessels (angiogenesis), which is when tumors need to grow and spread. They block the VEGF (vascular endothelial growth factor) pathway, preventing the formation of new blood vessels that supply oxygen and nutrients to tumors, thereby starving the cancer cells. *Examples*: Bevacizumab (Avastin), Sorafenib, Sunitinib.

Advantages of targeted Therapy: It has fewer side effects than chemotherapy, as it is more selective in its action.

Disadvantages: Targeted therapies may not work for all types of cancer, and cancer cells can sometimes develop resistance over time.

Immunotherapy

Immunotherapy is a treatment that boosts the body's natural defenses to fight cancer. It involves stimulating the immune system to recognize and attack cancer cells more effectively. Immunotherapy can involve using substances made by the body or in a laboratory to boost the immune system, making it more effective at identifying and destroying cancer cells.

Checkpoint Inhibitors:

One of the primary mechanisms of immunotherapy is through checkpoint inhibitors. Cancer cells often use certain proteins, such as PD-1 or CTLA-4, to 'turn off' immune cells and avoid detection. Checkpoint inhibitors block these proteins, allowing the immune system to recognize and attack cancer cells more effectively.

Examples include *Pembrolizumab and Nivolumab*, which are used in cancers such as melanoma, lung cancer, and kidney cancer.

Advantages of immunotherapy:

Immunotherapy can be very effective for certain cancers, such as melanoma and lung cancer, and can lead to long-term remission.

Disadvantages of immunotherapy:

Immunotherapy can have side effects, including flu-like symptoms, fatigue, and inflammation. Not all cancers respond to immunotherapy, and its effectiveness may take time to determine.

Hormone Therapy

Hormone therapy is used to treat cancers that are sensitive to hormones, such as breast and prostate cancers. The goal is to block the body's ability to produce the hormones that fuel the growth of these cancers or interfere with how the hormones work. Hormone therapy may involve medications that lower hormone levels or surgery to remove hormone-producing organs. *Examples: Anastrozole, letrozole, Exemestane*

Hormone therapy provides drugs that

- Block the effect of estrogen on breast cancer cells but may act like estrogen in other tissues. Examples: *Tamoxifen and raloxifene*

- Lower the level of estrogen in postmenopausal women by blocking the enzyme aromatase, which converts androgens to estrogen. Examples: Anastrozole, Letrozole, and Exemestane

- Block and degrade estrogen receptors in breast cancer cells. Example: *Fulvestrant (Faslodex)*.

- Lower estrogen levels by preventing the ovaries from producing estrogen, essentially causing temporary menopause.

- Lower testosterone levels by stopping the testicles from producing it (LHRH Agonists)

- Lower testosterone without the initial testosterone flare seen with LHRH agonists (LHRH Antagonists)

- Block androgen receptors on prostate cancer cells, preventing them from using testosterone.

- Block enzymes required for androgen production, reducing androgen levels.

- Slow the growth of endometrial cancer using synthetic forms of the hormone progesterone.

- Modulate estrogen activity

Advantages:

It can be effective in slowing or stopping the growth of hormone-sensitive cancers and can be used in conjunction with other treatments.

Disadvantages:

Side effects can include weight gain, mood changes, and changes in libido. It may not be suitable for cancers that do not respond to hormonal changes.

Combination Therapy

Combination therapy involves using two or more types of treatments to improve outcomes. For instance, a patient might undergo surgery to remove a tumor, followed by chemotherapy to kill any remaining cancer cells. This approach can maximize the chances of successful treatment.

Advantages:

Combining different treatments can attack cancer in multiple ways, increasing the likelihood of remission.

Disadvantages:

Combining therapies can also lead to increased side effects, as each treatment comes with its risks and challenges.

Managing Side Effects

Each of the conventional cancer treatments discussed above has potential side effects that can impact a patient's quality of life. Effective management of side effects is crucial to helping patients stay on track with their treatment plans.

Common Side Effects:

These may include fatigue, nausea, hair loss, loss of appetite, and weakened immune function.

Supportive Care:

Medications, dietary changes, physical activity, and complementary therapies can all help manage the side effects of cancer treatment.

Summary

Conventional cancer treatments are the cornerstone of cancer care and have been proven effective in numerous clinical trials. Depending on the type and Stage of cancer, different treatments or a combination may be recommended to achieve the best possible outcome. In the next chapter, we will look at the standard treatments for common cancers, exploring specific approaches for different cancer types and how these treatments are tailored to provide the best outcomes.

References:

1. National Cancer Institute. (2021). Types of Cancer Treatment. Retrieved from https://www.cancer.gov/about-cancer/treatme

nt/types

2. American Cancer Society. (2022). Understanding Cancer Treatment. Retrieved from https://www.cancer.org/treatment/treatments-and-side-effects.html

3. World Health Organization (WHO). (2022). Cancer Treatment Guidelines. Retrieved from https://www.who.int/health-topics/cancer/diagnosis-and-treatment

4. Mayo Clinic. (2021). Cancer Treatment: Overview of Options. Retrieved from https://www.mayoclinic.org/tests-procedures/cancer-treatment/about/pac-20393344

5. American Society of Clinical Oncology (ASCO). (2021). Cancer Treatment and Side Effects. Retrieved from https://www.cancer.net

Chapter 4

Standard Treatment of Common Cancers

In this chapter, we will explore the standard treatments for the most common types of cancer, including breast, lung, prostate, colorectal, liver, gastric, pancreatic, skin, and brain cancers. We will provide some statistics for each type of cancer, describe the drugs commonly used (grouped by their mechanism of action), and outline the treatment protocols for different stages. We will also discuss the effectiveness of these treatments based on five-year survival rates.

Breast Cancer

Breast cancer is the most common cancer among women globally, with approximately 2.3 million new cases diagnosed annually. The overall five-year survival rate for all breast cancer stages combined is around 90%, reflecting the fact that most breast cancers are diagnosed at earlier stages when the prognosis is better. However, the survival rates can vary based on tumor biology, hormone receptor status (ER/PR), HER2 status, and patient factors like age and overall health. While the five-year survival rate is nearly 100% in stage 0, it drops to as low as 30% in patients with metastatic breast cancer.

Therefore, it is important to act before a diagnosis can be made when we see any of the following early symptoms.

- Lump or thickening in the breast or underarm.
- Changes in breast shape or size.
- Nipple discharge, especially if it's bloody.
- Redness or dimpling of the skin on the breast (like an orange peel).
- Inverted nipple or changes in the nipple's appearance.

Conventional treatments for breast cancer vary depending on the Stage and specific characteristics of the cancer (e.g., hormone receptor status, HER2 status).

Treatment protocols by Stage of cancer

Stage I: Surgery (often lumpectomy) combined with radiation is highly effective. Hormone therapy or chemotherapy may be used depending on the cancer's molecular features.

Stage II: Surgery, often with chemotherapy and radiation, provides excellent outcomes. Targeted Therapy is used if HER2-positive. Hormone therapy is used for ER/PR-positive cancers.

Stage III: Requires a combination of surgery, chemotherapy, radiation, and targeted Therapy (if applicable). The goal is to control the tumor and reduce recurrence.

Stage IV: Treatment focuses on controlling the disease, prolonging life, and relieving symptoms. Chemotherapy, hormone therapy, targeted Therapy, and immunotherapy are commonly used.

Below are the common types of therapies in detail, with the types of surgery and drugs to be used for different stages of cancer and the potential side effects:

1. Surgery

- **Lumpectomy**: This involves removing the tumor and a small margin of surrounding tissue. It is usually followed by radiation.

- **Mastectomy**: Removal of the entire breast. In some cases, both breasts may be removed (double mastectomy).

- **Lymph Node Dissection**: If cancer has spread to the lymph nodes, some or all of the lymph nodes in the underarm area may be removed.

3. Chemotherapy

- It can be given before surgery (neoadjuvant chemotherapy) to shrink tumors or after surgery (adjuvant chemotherapy) to kill remaining cancer cells.

- Common drugs include anthracyclines (doxorubicin), taxanes (paclitaxel), platinum-based drugs (Carboplatin), Tamoxifen, anastrozole, and letrozole, and Cyclophosphamide.

4. Hormone (Endocrine) Therapy

Tamoxifen: Blocks estrogen receptors on cancer cells. **Aromatase Inhibitors (AIs):** Reduce estrogen production (e.g., *letrozole, anastrozole*). And **Ovarian Suppression:** For premenopausal women, medications (or surgery) to shut down the ovaries may be used. e.g. *leuprolite (Lupron) or goserelin (Zoladex)*

5. Targeted Therapy

HER2-Targeted Therapies: Trastuzumab (Herceptin), pertuzumab, and others target the HER2 protein, which is overexpressed in some breast cancers. **CDK4/6 Inhibitors**: Palbociclib and ribociclib are used in combination with hormone therapy to slow cancer growth. **PARP Inhibitors**: Olaparib, used for patients with BRCA1/2 mutations.

6. Immunotherapy

Commonly used Drugs: **Checkpoint Inhibitor**s (e.g., pembrolizumab) for triple-negative breast cancer that expresses PD-L1.

Lung Cancer

Lung cancer is one of the leading causes of cancer-related deaths worldwide, with about 2.2 million new cases each year. The five-year survival rate for non-small cell lung cancer (NSCLC) is 26%, while for small cell lung cancer (SCLC), it is only around 7%. However, treatment from stage 1 may result in an 80% five-year survival rate. It is, therefore, very beneficial to act before being able to secure a diagnosis when we see any of the early symptoms:

Chronic cough or a cough that worsens over time., – Coughing up blood (hemoptysis), – Shortness of breath or wheezing.- Chest pain that may worsen with deep breathing or coughing.- Hoarseness or voice changes. – Frequent respiratory infections, like bronchitis or pneumonia.

Lung cancer treatment is highly dependent on the Stage and type of lung cancer (Non-Small Cell Lung Cancer [NSCLC] or Small Cell Lung Cancer [SCLC]).

Treatment protocols by Stage of cancer

Stage I (Early-Stage NSCLC): Surgery or SBRT is highly effective, often with a curative intent. If the tumor is more extensive or aggressive, chemotherapy may follow. The five-year survival rate is around 80%.

Stage II (Locally Advanced NSCLC): Adjuvant chemotherapy typically follows surgery to improve survival. In some cases, radiation is added if surgery is not an option—a five-year survival rate of around 60%.

Stage III (Locally Advanced NSCLC): Chemoradiation is the standard treatment. Surgery may be considered in select cases, but chemotherapy and radiation are often combined to reduce tumor size and prevent spread. The five-year survival rate is around 30%.

Stage IV (Metastatic NSCLC/SCLC): Treatment focuses on controlling the disease and prolonging life. Based on the cancer's molecular profile, chemotherapy, immunotherapy, and targeted therapies are used. Surgery is typically an option for palliative reasons. The five-year survival rate is around 6%.

Below are the common types of therapies in detail, with the types of surgery and drugs to be used for different stages of cancer and the potential side effects:

1. Surgery

Types:

- **Lobectomy**: Removal of an entire lobe of the lung (most common).

- **Pneumonectomy**: Removal of an entire lung.

- **Segmentectomy/Wedge Resection**: This procedure removes part of a lobe. It is typically used in early-stage cancers when a smaller portion can be removed.

2. Radiation Therapy

- External Beam Radiation: Delivers high-energy rays to the tumor from outside the body.

- Stereotactic Body Radiation Therapy (SBRT): A highly focused form of radiation used for small, early-stage tumors.

- Prophylactic Cranial Irradiation (PCI): Used in SCLC to prevent cancer from spreading to the brain.

3. Chemotherapy

Types of drugs:

- Common drugs include platinum-based compounds (cisplatin or Carboplatin) combined with others like paclitaxel, vinorelbine, or etoposide. Cisplatin and carboplatin are platinum-based compounds that cross-link DNA and induce oxidative stress, which leads to cancer cell death. Paclitaxel is a microtubule inhibitor used to disrupt the microtubules critical for cell division. It causes cancer cells to stop dividing and eventually die. Etoposide is a topoisomerase inhibitor that prevents DNA unwinding, thereby halting cell division and inducing apoptosis.

4. Targeted Therapy

Types of drugs:

- Erlotinib and Osimertinib. Erlotinib is a tyrosine kinase inhibitor (TKI) that targets the epidermal growth factor receptor (EGFR) pathway, which is overactive in some lung cancers. By inhibiting this pathway, erlotinib effectively blocks cell proliferation. Osimertinib is another TKI that specifically targets EGFR mutations, particularly the T790M mutation, which is associated with resistance to other EGFR inhibitors.

- Alectinib, Crizotinib, and other drugs target anaplastic lymphoma kinase (ALK) gene mutations, inhibiting proteins involved in the abnormal growth of tumor cells.

- Other Targeted Drugs: Target mutations like ROS1, BRAF, and MET, as well as angiogenesis (e.g., bevacizumab).

5. Immunotherapy

- Checkpoint Inhibitors: Pembrolizumab (Keytruda), nivolumab (Opdivo), and atezolizumab (Tecentriq) help the immune system recognize and attack cancer cells.

- PD-1/PD-L1 Inhibitors: These drugs block proteins that prevent the immune system from attacking cancer cells.

6. Chemoradiation (Combination of Chemotherapy and Radiation)

Often used in Stage III NSCLC and limited-stage SCLC. It combines the strengths of both treatments to shrink the tumor before surgery or as the primary treatment in patients who are not surgical candidates.

Prostate Cancer

Prostate cancer is the second most common cancer among men, with around 1.4 million cases diagnosed annually. The five-year survival rate for early-stage prostate cancer is nearly 100% but drops significantly to about 30% for metastatic Stage. The overall five-year survival rate for all stages of prostate cancer combined is close to 98-99% due to the effectiveness of treatment in the early stages. It is, therefore, beneficial to act before being able to secure a diagnosis appointment when we see any of the following early symptoms: -Difficulty urinating (weak stream, frequent urination, especially at night).- Pain or burning sensation during urination.- Blood in the urine or semen.- Erectile dysfunction.- Pain in the hips, back, or pelvis (may indicate cancer has spread).

Prostate cancer treatment depends on the Stage of cancer, the patient's health, and the aggressiveness of the cancer. Common conventional therapies include surgery, radiation therapy, hormone therapy, chemotherapy, and, in some cases, targeted Therapy or immunotherapy.

Treatment protocols by Stage of cancer

The effectiveness varies depending on the Stage of cancer at which treatment starts. Prostate cancer generally has a high five-year survival rate, especially when detected early.

Stage I (Localized): Surgery or radiation therapy is often curative. Active surveillance is an option for men with very low-risk, slow-growing cancer. The prognosis is excellent, with high five-year survival rates of nearly 100%

Stage II (Localized but more advanced): Surgery and radiation are still highly effective, especially when combined with hormone therapy in some cases. Cure rates remain high with aggressive treatment, with five-year survival rates of nearly 100%

Stage III (Locally Advanced): A combination of radiation and hormone therapy is typically used. Surgery may still be an option in some cases. Treatment at this Stage is aimed at controlling cancer and preventing further spread. The five-year survival rate remains high, around 95-100%, especially with aggressive treatment.

Stage IV (Metastatic): Treatment focuses on slowing progression, managing symptoms, and extending survival. Hormone therapy, chemotherapy, targeted Therapy, and immunotherapy are used, but these are not curative. The five-year survival rate drop significantly to about 30% as the cancer has spread to other parts of the body. However, some men with advanced disease live longer with treatment advancements.

Below are detailed therapies, including commonly used drugs and their side effects.

1. Surgery

Radical Prostatectomy is the most common surgery for localized prostate cancer. It involves removing the prostate gland, seminal vesicles, and sometimes nearby lymph nodes. It can be done through open surgery or minimally invasive laparoscopic/robot-assisted methods.

2. Radiation Therapy

- **External Beam Radiation Therapy (EBRT):** High-energy X-rays are directed at the prostate to kill cancer cells.

- **Brachytherapy (Internal Radiation):** Radioactive seeds or pellets are implanted into the prostate to deliver radiation directly to the cancer.

3. Hormone Therapy (Androgen Deprivation Therapy, ADT)

- **LHRH Agonists/Antagonists:** Drugs like leuprolide, goserelin, and degarelix reduce testosterone production by the testicles, slowing cancer growth.

- **Anti-Androgens:** Drugs such as bicalutamide block the effect of testosterone on prostate cancer cells.

4. Chemotherapy

Types of drugs

Docetaxel and Cabazitaxel are common chemotherapy drugs used for prostate cancer, especially in advanced stages when hormone therapy is no longer effective. These work by disrupting microtubule assembly dynamics and inducing cell cycle arrest, ultimately triggering apoptosis.

5. Targeted Therapy

PARP Inhibitors: Olaparib and Rucaparib target cancer cells with specific genetic mutations (e.g., BRCA1 or BRCA2).

6. Immunotherapy

Sipuleucel-T (Provenge) is a therapeutic cancer vaccine that stimulates the immune system to attack prostate cancer cells.

7. Active Surveillance

For low-risk, slow-growing prostate cancers (especially in older men), active surveillance involves regular monitoring (PSA tests, biopsies, imaging) without immediate treatment.

Colorectal (Colon and Rectal) Cancer

Colorectal cancer is the third most common cancer globally, with over 1.9 million new cases each year. The five-year survival rate for localized colorectal cancer is around 90%, but it drops significantly to 11-14% for metastatic disease. It is, therefore, beneficial to act before being able to secure a diagnosis when we see more than one of the following early symptoms: – Changes in bowel habits, such as diarrhea, constipation, or narrowing of the stool.- Blood in the stool (either bright red or very dark). -Abdominal discomfort (cramping, pain, or bloating).- Unexplained weight loss.- Fatigue or weakness.

Colorectal cancer treatment depends on the Stage of the cancer, its location, and whether it has spread. Common treatments include surgery, chemotherapy, radiation therapy, and targeted Therapy.

Treatment protocols by Stage of cancer.

Stage 0 (Carcinoma in situ): Surgery is highly effective, with almost all patients being cured.

Stage I: Surgery alone is often curative, with a very high success rate (90%+ five-year survival rate).

Stage II: Surgery is the primary treatment, and chemotherapy may be added in high-risk cases. About 75-85% of patients survive five years or more.

Stage III: Surgery combined with chemotherapy improves survival. Depending on lymph node involvement, the five-year survival rate ranges from 50% to 75%.

Stage IV: While cure is rare, treatment focuses on extending life and managing symptoms. Targeted therapies and immunotherapies can be very effective for certain patients. The five-year survival rate is around 11-14%, though it varies widely depending on the extent of metastasis and response to treatment.

Below are detailed descriptions of therapies used in the treatment of colorectal cancer, including commonly used drugs and their side effects.

1. Surgery

Polypectomy and Local Excision: For very early-stage cancer (Stage 0 or I), polyps or small tumors can be removed during a colonoscopy.

Colectomy (Colon Resection): Removing part or all of the colon, along with nearby lymph nodes.

Colostomy or Ileostomy: In some cases, part of the bowel may be diverted to an external bag to allow healing.

2. Chemotherapy

- Common drugs include fluorouracil (5-FU), capecitabine, oxaliplatin, and irinotecan.

- 5-FU and capecitabine are antimetabolite drugs that block cancer cells' ability to make copies of DNA and divide.

- Irinotecan blocks topoisomerase enzyme to prevent cancer cells from dividing.

- Oxaliplatin is an alkylating agent that damages cell DNA, stops or slows the growth of cancer cells and other rapidly growing cells, and causes them to die.

- Adjuvant chemotherapy: Given after surgery to eliminate remaining cancer cells and reduce recurrence.

- Neoadjuvant chemotherapy: Given before surgery to shrink tumors.

3. Radiation Therapy

- **External Beam Radiation Therapy:** High-energy X-rays target the cancer from outside the body.

- **Internal Radiation (Brachytherapy):** Rarely used, but small radioactive pellets can be placed near the tumor.

4. Targeted Therapy

- **EGFR (Epidermal growth factor receptor) Inhibitors**: Cetuximab and Panitumumab target EGFR mutations in cancer cells.

- **VEGF Inhibitors:** Bevacizumab targets blood vessel growth in the tumor (anti-angiogenesis).

- **Immunotherapy:** Pembrolizumab and nivolumab are used for MSI-H (microsatellite instability-high) cancers.

5. Immunotherapy

Checkpoint inhibitors like Pembrolizumab or Nivolumab are used for advanced cancers that are MSI-H or dMMR (deficient mismatch repair).

Liver Cancer

Liver cancer accounts for over 800,000 new cases globally each year, with a low five-year survival rate of around 20% due to late diagnosis but as low as 3% for metastatic Stage. It is, therefore, beneficial to act before being able to secure a diagnosis appointment when we see more than one of the following early symptoms: – Unexplained weight loss. -Loss of appetite or feeling full quickly.- Abdominal pain or swelling, especially in the upper right quadrant.- Yellowing of the skin and eyes (jaundice).- Nausea and vomiting. -General fatigue and weakness.

Liver cancer (hepatocellular carcinoma or HCC) treatment depends on factors such as the Stage of the cancer, the size and number of tumors, liver function, and the patient's overall health. Common conventional therapies include surgery, ablation, embolization, radiation therapy, targeted Therapy, immunotherapy, and chemotherapy.

Treatment protocols by Stage of cancer:

Stage I: Localized (confined to the liver): Surgical resection, ablation, or liver transplant. The five-year survival rate is about 35%

Stage II-(localized advanced cancer): Surgery or transplant, ablation, and embolization.

Stage III: Regional (spread to nearby tissues or lymph nodes): Targeted Therapy, Immunotherapy, Radiation therapy. The five-year survival rate is around 12%

Stage IV: Distant (metastatic, spread to distant organs): Targeted Therapy and Immunotherapy are used. The five-year survival rate is around 3%

These survival rates are influenced by factors like liver function (e.g., the presence of cirrhosis), treatment response, and the patient's general health.

Below are detailed descriptions of the therapies for liver cancer, including the types of radiation, commonly used drugs, and their side effects:

1. Surgery

- **Partial Hepatectomy:** Removal of part of the liver containing the tumor.

- **Liver Transplant:** Replacing the entire liver with a healthy liver from a donor.

2. Ablation

Ablation is a way to destroy the tumor by applying heat or cold directly to it.

- **Radiofrequency Ablation (RFA):** Uses high-energy radio waves to heat and destroy cancer cells.

- **Microwave Ablation:** Destroys cancer using microwave energy.

- **Cryoablation**: Freezes cancer cells.

3. Embolization

Embolization is a procedure in which substances are injected directly into the hepatic artery of the liver. The goal is to block or reduce blood flow to a tumor in the liver.

- **Trans-arterial Chemoembolization (TACE):** Chemotherapy

is directly delivered to the tumor through a catheter into the hepatic artery, and the blood supply to the tumor is blocked.

- **Radioembolizations (Y90):** Tiny radioactive beads are injected into the liver to target cancer cells.

- **Trans-arterial Embolization (TAE):** Embolization without chemotherapy or radiation but with small particles into the artery to plug it up, preventing key nutrients and oxygen from going to the tumor.

4. Radiation Therapy

- **External Beam Radiation Therapy (EBRT):** Uses high-energy rays to target liver tumors.

- **Stereotactic Body Radiation Therapy (SBRT):** Delivers very precise, high doses of radiation to the tumor.

5. Targeted Therapy

Common drugs:

- Sorafenib (Nexavar) and Lenvatinib (Lenvima): Block cancer cell growth and blood vessel formation.

- Regorafenib (Stivarga) and Cabozantinib (Cabometyx): Used in advanced liver cancer.

6. Immunotherapy

- Atezolizumab (Tecentriq) with Bevacizumab (Avastin): A combination approved for advanced liver cancer.

- Nivolumab (Opdivo): A checkpoint inhibitor used in advanced liver cancer.

7. Chemotherapy

Chemotherapy is used less frequently in liver cancer, as it is often ineffective compared to other treatments

- Traditional chemotherapy is not as effective for liver cancer as it is for other types of cancer.

- It is generally used only if targeted therapies or immunotherapies are not working.

Gastric or Stomach Cancer

Gastric cancer accounts for over one million new cases each year. The five-year survival rate varies significantly, from 70% for localized cancer to less than 6% for advanced cancer. It is, therefore, beneficial to act before being able to secure a diagnosis when we see one or more of the following early symptoms: -Indigestion or persistent heartburn.- Feeling bloated after eating, even a small meal.- Nausea or vomiting (sometimes with blood).- Unexplained weight loss.- Abdominal pain, especially after eating.

Gastric cancer, or stomach cancer, is often diagnosed in later stages, which impacts the effectiveness of treatment. The main conventional therapies include surgery, chemotherapy, radiation therapy, and, in some cases, targeted therapies. The approach depends on the cancer's Stage, location, and the patient's overall health.

Treatment protocol by Stage of cancer

Stage I (Localized): Surgery offers the best chance for a cure, with a high five-year survival rate (65-80%) if the cancer is detected early and confined to the stomach lining. Chemotherapy or radiation may follow surgery.

Stage II (Locally Advanced): Surgery, combined with chemotherapy and radiation, remains the standard treatment. The chance of recurrence is higher, but aggressive treatment can still lead to long-term survival (30-40% five years)

Stage III (Advanced): Surgery may still be an option, often followed by chemoradiation. However, the prognosis worsens as the cancer spreads to nearby lymph nodes and organs. Chemotherapy is often used before or after surgery. The five-year survival rate drops to 10-20%

Stage IV (Metastatic): Surgery is rarely curative, and treatment focuses on chemotherapy, targeted Therapy, or immunotherapy to slow disease progression and manage symptoms. The goal is to extend life and improve quality of life, but the cancer is typically not curable at this Stage. The five-year survival rate is low, around 4-6%.

The overall five-year survival rate for all stages combined is approximately 32%. Early detection significantly improves outcomes, but many cases are diagnosed at more advanced stages.

Following are all the therapies used for gastric cancer in detail, including commonly used surgeries, drugs, radiation, and their side effects.

1. Surgery

- **Subtotal (Partial) Gastrectomy:** This procedure removes part of the stomach, typically for cancers located in the lower part of the stomach.

- **Total Gastrectomy:** This procedure removes the entire stomach, often for larger tumors or those in the upper part of the stomach.

- **Lymphadenectomy**: Removal of nearby lymph nodes is standard during surgery to check for cancer spread.

2. Chemotherapy

- Common drugs include 5-fluorouracil (5-FU), Cisplatin, Capecitabine, Oxaliplatin, and Irinotecan.

- **Neoadjuvant chemotherapy**: Administered before surgery to shrink the tumor and improve surgical outcomes.

- **Adjuvant chemotherapy:** Given after surgery to kill any remaining cancer cells and reduce recurrence risk.

3. Radiation Therapy

External Beam Radiation Therapy (EBRT): Focuses high-energy X-rays on the tumor site.

4. Targeted Therapy

Commonly used drugs:

- **Trastuzumab (Herceptin):** Used for gastric cancers that overexpress the HER2 protein, often in combination with chemotherapy for advanced-stage cancers.

- **Ramucirumab (Cyramza):** An anti-angiogenesis drug that targets blood vessel growth in tumors, used for advanced cancers that are no longer responding to chemotherapy.

- **Pembrolizumab (Keytruda):** An immune checkpoint inhibitor used for advanced gastric cancers with high microsatellite instability (MSI-H) or PD-L1 expression.

5. Immunotherapy

Pembrolizumab (Keytruda): Approved for advanced or metastatic gastric cancer that has specific genetic mutations (MSI-H or PD-L1-positive).

Pancreatic Cancer

Pancreatic cancer is one of the deadliest cancers, with over 460,000 cases annually. The overall five-year survival rate for all stages of pancreatic cancer is approximately 12%, ranging from 39% down to 1% from early Stage to advanced Stage. Early detection and surgery provide the best chances for long-term survival, but unfortunately, most cases are diagnosed at later stages. It is, therefore, important to act before being able to secure a diagnosis when we notice one or more of the following early symptoms:- Jaundice (yellowing of the skin and eyes). – Dark urine and pale stools.- Abdominal or back pain that may radiate to the back.- Unexplained weight loss.- Loss of appetite.- New onset of diabetes (rising blood sugar level) or worsening of existing diabetes.

Pancreatic cancer is particularly aggressive and challenging to treat due to late diagnosis and rapid progression. The main conventional therapies include surgery, chemotherapy, radiation therapy, and, in some cases, targeted therapies. The treatment approach depends on the Stage of the cancer and the patient's overall health.

Treatment Protocols by Stage of Cancer

Stage I (Localized): Surgery is the primary curative option. If the cancer is localized and the patient is healthy enough for surgery, the prognosis improves. Chemotherapy and sometimes radiation may follow surgery to reduce the risk of recurrence.

Stage II (Locally advanced): Surgery is still possible, and chemotherapy or radiation is often used to increase the chances of successful removal. Treatment can improve survival, but recurrence is common.

Stage III (Unresectable, Locally Advanced): Surgery is usually not possible, and treatment focuses on chemotherapy, radiation, or both to control the disease and prolong survival. It is not typically curative at this Stage.

Stage IV (Metastatic): Surgery is not an option, and the focus is on chemotherapy, targeted Therapy, or immunotherapy (for specific genetic profiles). Treatment can help extend life and manage symptoms, but it is not curative.

The following are the therapies for pancreatic cancer in detail, including commonly used surgeries, radiation, and drugs, as well as their side effects.

1. Surgery

- **Whipple Procedure (Pancreaticoduodenectomy):** This surgery removes the head of the pancreas, part of the small intestine, bile duct, and sometimes part of the stomach. It is the most common surgery for tumors in the head of the pancreas.

- **Distal Pancreatectomy:** Removes the tail of the pancreas and possibly the spleen.

- **Total Pancreatectomy:** This procedure removes the entire pancreas, part of the stomach, small intestine, bile duct, and spleen.

2. Chemotherapy

Common Drugs:

- FOLFIRINOX (a combination of 5-fluorouracil, leucovorin, irinotecan, and oxaliplatin) is one of the most effective chemotherapy regimens for pancreatic cancer, often used for patients in good health.

- Gemcitabine (alone or in combination with Abraxane) is commonly used, especially for patients who cannot tolerate more aggressive chemotherapy like FOLFIRINOX.

- Capecitabine, – Cisplatin- Irinotecan- Oxaliplatin- Nab-paclitaxel

3. Radiation Therapy

- **External Beam Radiation Therapy (EBRT):** Uses high-energy X-rays to target the tumor.

- **Stereotactic Body Radiation Therapy (SBRT):** It is a more precise, high-dose form of radiation therapy used for certain patients.

4. Targeted Therapy

- **Erlotinib (Tarceva)**: Used for advanced pancreatic cancer in combination with gemcitabine. It targets the epidermal growth factor receptor (EGFR), which helps cancer cells grow.

- **Larotrectinib or Entrectinib:** Used in rare cases of pancreatic cancer with specific gene mutations (NTRK gene fusions).

5. Immunotherapy (Limited Use)

Pembrolizumab (Keytruda): An immune checkpoint inhibitor approved for patients with pancreatic cancer that has certain genetic changes (microsatellite instability-high, or MSI-H).

Skin Cancer (Melanoma)

Melanoma accounts for over 300,000 new cases annually. The five-year survival rate is about 92% for localized melanoma but drops to 30% for advanced stages. It is, therefore, always beneficial to act before securing a diagnosis when we see one or more of the following early symptoms:- Changes in moles (size, shape, color, or texture).- New skin growths or sores that do not heal.- Itching, tenderness, or pain around a mole or spot.- Dark streaks under nails. -Unexplained bleeding from a mole.

Melanoma, a serious form of skin cancer, is treatable, especially if detected early. Conventional treatments include surgery, radiation therapy, chemotherapy, targeted Therapy, and immunotherapy. The choice of Therapy depends on the cancer stage, tumor thickness, and whether the melanoma has spread to other parts of the body.

Treatment protocols by Stage of cancer

Stage 0 (In Situ): Surgery (wide local excision) is typically curative and has an excellent prognosis. With early detection and surgical removal, the five-year survival rate is almost 100%.

Stage I (Localized): Surgery remains highly effective, with a cure rate of more than 90% for early-stage melanoma. The five-year survival rate is around 90-95%, as the cancer is still localized to the skin.

Stage II (Localized but High Risk): Surgery is the main treatment, but there is a higher risk of recurrence. Additional treatments like adjuvant immunotherapy may be considered in some cases. The five-year survival rate drops to 70-80% as the tumor is thicker and more likely to spread.

Stage III (Regional Spread): Surgery, often followed by adjuvant therapies like immunotherapy or targeted Therapy, is used. The risk of recurrence is higher, but modern treatments significantly improve outcomes. The five-year survival rate is 40-70%, depending on the extent of spread to lymph nodes.

Stage IV (Metastatic): Melanoma that has spread to distant organs is more challenging to treat. Immunotherapy, targeted Therapy, or a combination of both can control the disease and improve survival, though the cancer is generally not curable at this Stage. The five-year survival rate for metastatic melanoma is about 15-25%. However, advances in immunotherapy and targeted Therapy have improved survival in recent years, with some patients experiencing long-term remission.

The following are the therapies for Skin cancer in detail, including the types of surgery, radiation, and commonly used drugs and their side effects.

1. Surgery

- **Wide Local Excision:** This involves removing the melanoma along with a margin of healthy tissue around it. It is the most common treatment for early-stage melanoma.

- **Sentinel Lymph Node Biopsy:** Removal of nearby lymph nodes to check for cancer spread.

- **Lymphadenectomy:** Removal of lymph nodes if cancer has spread to them.

2. Radiation Therapy

External Beam Radiation Therapy (EBRT): High-energy X-rays target the melanoma site to destroy cancer cells.

3. Chemotherapy

Common drugs include Dacarbazine (DTIC), Temozolomide, and combinations like Cisplatin and Vinblastine.

4. Targeted Therapy

Drugs that target specific mutations in melanoma cells, such as BRAF inhibitors (Vemurafenib, Dabrafenib) and MEK inhibitors (Trametinib, Cobimetinib), are effective for melanomas with BRAF mutations (present in about 50% of cases).

5. Immunotherapy

- **Checkpoint Inhibitors:** Drugs like Pembrolizumab (Keytruda), Nivolumab (Opdivo), and Ipilimumab (Yervoy) stimulate the immune system to attack melanoma cells.

- **Interleukin-2 (IL-2):** A drug that boosts immune cell activity to fight

6. Targeted Radiation (Stereotactic Radiosurgery)

Stereotactic Body Radiation Therapy (SBRT) or Stereotactic Radiosurgery (SRS): These methods deliver precise, high-dose radiation to small tumors, especially in the brain.

Brain Cancer (Glioblastoma)

Glioblastoma is the most aggressive form of brain cancer, with about 250,000 new cases each year. The five-year survival rate is less than 7%. It is, therefore, crucial to act before being able to secure a diagnosis when we see one or more of the following early symptoms: – Headaches that become more frequent or severe. – Seizures.- Nausea or vomiting- Vision problems (blurred vision, double vision).- Difficulty with balance or speech. – Changes in personality or behavior. -Weakness or numbness in one side of the body.

Glioblastoma (GBM) is an aggressive and difficult-to-treat brain cancer. Treatment aims to slow its progression, relieve symptoms, and prolong survival, as glioblastoma is not curable. Conventional therapies include surgery, radiation therapy, chemotherapy, and sometimes newer treatments like targeted therapies.

Treatment Protocol by Stage of Cancer

Stage I-II (Low-Grade Glioma): Glioblastoma is rarely detected at these stages because it grows aggressively. In cases where lower -grade gliomas transform into glioblastoma, surgery followed by radiation and chemotherapy is the primary approach, but survival outcomes vary.

Stage III (Localized but Advanced): Surgery followed by radiation and chemotherapy can prolong survival, but recurrence is common. Glioblastoma spreads rapidly and infiltrates surrounding brain tissue, making complete removal is difficult.

Stage IV (Advanced/Metastatic): Glioblastoma is highly aggressive at this Stage. The goal of treatment is to manage symptoms, slow progression, and extend life. The combination of surgery, radiation, chemotherapy, and sometimes tumor-treating fields can improve survival but not cure the disease.

Median survival is about 14-16 months for patients in Stages III and IV undergoing surgery, radiation, and chemotherapy. Some patients treated with Optune or bevacizumab may live longer, but survival beyond two years is rare.

Following are the therapies for brain cancer in detail, including the types of surgery, radiation, commonly used drugs, and their side effects.

1. Surgery

- **Craniotomy with Tumor Resection:** The main surgery for glioblastoma is to remove as much of the tumor as possible. Complete removal is often challenging due to the tumor's infiltration into nearby brain tissue.

- Surgery improves symptoms and quality of life but is not curative, as glioblastoma typically returns even after maximal tumor resection.

2. Radiation Therapy

- **External Beam Radiation Therapy (EBRT):** Standard radiation therapy is often combined with chemotherapy after surgery. Radiation is delivered to the tumor site and surrounding brain tissue.

- **Stereotactic Radiosurgery (SRS):** A more focused, high-dose form of radiation, sometimes used for recurrent glioblastoma or in combination with surgery.

Glioblastoma is highly resistant to radiation, but it can reduce the tumor's growth and improve survival by several months.

3. Chemotherapy

- **Temozolomide (Temodar):** The most commonly used chemotherapy drug for glioblastoma, often administered alongside radiation therapy and afterward as part of maintenance therapy.

- Chemotherapy is often less effective for glioblastoma than other cancers because many drugs cannot cross the blood-brain barrier.

4. Tumor Treating Fields (Optune)

This is a wearable device that uses electrical fields to disrupt cancer cell division and slow the tumor's growth. It is used in combination with chemotherapy (Temozolomide).

While not curative, it may prolong progression-free and overall survival in some patients.

5. Targeted Therapy

- **Bevacizumab (Avastin):** A targeted therapy that inhibits the growth of blood vessels (anti-angiogenesis Therapy) to the tumor, slowing its progression.

It does not cure glioblastoma but can reduce tumor growth and alleviate symptoms.

6. Immunotherapy

- **Checkpoint Inhibitors:** Due to the brain's immune-suppressive environment, drugs like pembrolizumab have shown limited success in glioblastoma.

- Immunotherapy has not become standard for glioblastoma due to the tumor's resistance to immune response.

Questions to ask your oncologist/ doctors

- What are the standard treatment options for my specific type and Stage of cancer?

- What is the goal of each recommended treatment? (e.g., cure, control, symptom relief)

- What are the potential side effects of the chemotherapy, targeted Therapy and immunotherapy drugs being suggested?

- What are the success rates of the recommended treatments, particularly in terms of five-year survival?

- Can we discuss how to combine well-researched complementary therapies that may enhance the effectiveness and reduce the side effects of conventional treatment?

- What lifestyle changes (diet, exercise, stress management) should I make to support my treatment? Can we discuss this?

Summary

Standard treatments for common cancers vary significantly depending on the type and Stage of the disease. Most of them are effective at the earliest Stage of cancer. It is, therefore, very important to act when early symptoms appear before diagnosis. Understanding these treatments and their effectiveness helps in making informed decisions about care options. In the next chapter, we will explore the role of natural and complementary therapies, as well as their potential benefits and challenges in cancer care.

References:

1. National Cancer Institute (NCI). (2022). Types of Cancer Treatment by Cancer Type. Retrieved from https://www.cancer.gov/types

2. American Cancer Society (ACS). (2021). Cancer Treatment by Type and Stage. Retrieved from https://www.cancer.org/treatment/treatments-and-side-effects

3. Mayo Clinic. (2022). Cancer Treatment Options for Different Cancer Types. Retrieved from https://www.mayoclinic.org/diseases-conditions/cancer/diagnosis-treatment

4. World Health Organization (WHO). (2022). Cancer Diagnosis and Treatment Guide. Retrieved from https://www.who.int/health-topics/cancer/diagnosis-and-treatment

5. American Society of Clinical Oncology (ASCO). (2021). Cancer Treatment Guides by Cancer Type. Retrieved from https://www.cancer.net/cancer-types

Chapter 5

Conventional Treatments Need Complementary Help

Why?

Conventional cancer treatments, such as chemotherapy and radiotherapy, are often the primary choice for managing and controlling cancer. However, these treatments face significant challenges, especially in advanced stages of cancer, which limits their effectiveness and necessitates complementary support. Some of the primary challenges include:

Drug Resistance: Over time, many cancer cells develop resistance to chemotherapy drugs, making them less effective or even ineffective. This resistance can occur due to various mechanisms, including changes in cancer cell genetics or enhanced drug efflux systems that remove drugs from the cells before they can act.

Cancer Cells' Insensitivity to Drugs: Cancer cells can sometimes become less sensitive to the effects of chemotherapy or radiation, reducing the overall efficacy of treatment. This insensitivity means that conventional drugs may need additional support to penetrate and impact cancer cells effectively.

Inability to Kill Cancer Stem Cells (CSCs): Conventional therapies often fail to completely eradicate cancer stem cells, which are a subset of cells capable of self-renewal and driving tumor regrowth. CSCs are resistant to standard treatments due to their robust DNA repair mechanisms and ability to remain in a quiescent state, making it difficult for chemotherapy or radiation to eliminate them entirely.

Inability to Stop Metastasis: One of the major challenges of conventional treatment is its inability to effectively prevent or stop metastasis—the spread of cancer cells to other parts of the body. Once metastasis occurs, cancer becomes significantly more difficult to manage, and standard therapies may not be sufficient to contain its spread.

Causing adverse side effects and wreaking havoc to patients' quality of life: Conventional cancer treatments, such as chemotherapy and radiotherapy, often pose significant challenges due to their severe adverse side effects. These therapies, while effective at targeting cancer cells, can also harm healthy tissues, leading to debilitating symptoms like fatigue, nausea, organ toxicity, immune suppression, and cognitive decline. Such side effects not only make the treatment process physically demanding but also have a profound impact on the patient's mental and emotional well-being, drastically diminishing their quality of life during and after treatment.

How Natural Therapies can help

Natural therapies can provide the complementary help needed to address these limitations. By targeting cancer stem cells, supporting immune function, reducing resistance, and enhancing the overall effectiveness of conventional treatments, these natural products offer a valuable addition to the cancer treatment arsenal.

Research and clinical studies show that common natural products such as Aloe Arborescens, Bitter melon, Black seeds, Blueberries, Flaxseeds, Fucoidan, Garlic, Ginger, Honey, Mistletoes, Papaya, Perilla, probiotics, Turmeric, Virgin Coconut Oil (VCO) can provide complementary help to enhance the effectiveness of conventional therapies and minimize their adverse side effects on patients. Apart from specific products used in natural therapies to complement cancer treatment, as listed below, adopting a healthy diet and lifestyle also provides essential natural support to conventional treatment. Chapters 8 and 9 will explain the role of diet and mind-body healing in cancer treatment.

The following table show the complementary effects the above natural products can have on conventional therapies.

Natural Products	Enhance Efficacy	Protect against Toxicity	Reduce side effects	Support Immune	Reduce Pain	Improve life quality	Support Detox	Anti Cancer
Aloe Arb.	✓	✓	✓	✓	✓	✓	✓	✓
Bitter melon	✓	✓	✓	✓	✓	✓		✓
Black seeds	✓	✓	✓	✓	✓	✓	✓	✓
Blueberries	✓		✓		✓			✓
fFlaxseeds	✓	✓	✓	✓	✓	✓	✓	✓
Fucoidan	✓		✓	✓	✓	✓		✓
Garlic	✓	✓	✓	✓	✓	✓	✓	✓
Ginger	✓		✓		✓	✓		✓
Honey	✓	✓	✓	✓	✓	✓		✓
Mistletoe			✓	✓	✓	✓		✓
Papaya	✓	✓	✓	✓	✓	✓	✓	✓
Perilla	✓	✓	✓	✓	✓	✓	✓	✓
Probiotics	✓	✓	✓	✓	✓	✓		✓
Turmeric	✓		✓	✓	✓			
Virgin Coconut Oil	✓	✓	✓	✓	✓	✓	✓	✓

Table 1: Common Natural Products that complement Standard Care

Common anti-cancer products in natural therapies

Following are summaries of the benefits to cancer treatment of Aloe Arborescens, Bitter Melon, Black Cumin, Blueberries, Flaxseeds, Fucoidan, Garlic, Ginger, Honey, Mistletoe, Papaya, Perilla, Probiotics & fermented foods, Turmeric and Virgin Coconut Oil. The details of these benefits including references and clinical evidence for each natural product are in the Appendices.

Aloe arborescens

Aloe arborescens is a succulent plant, closely related to Aloe vera, native to southern Africa. It has been used for centuries in traditional medicine for wound healing, skin conditions, and digestive issues. Recently, it has gained attention for its therapeutic properties, such as anti-inflammatory, antioxidant, immunomodulatory, anti-cancer, antibacterial, and detoxifying effects. For cancer treatment those plants aged over five years arev most suitable.

Benefits of Aloe arborescens in Cancer Treatment

Aloe arborescens has shown potential as a complementary therapy in cancer treatment, enhancing chemotherapy and radiotherapy, protecting against toxicity, and improving patients' quality of life.

Enhancement of Chemotherapy and Radiotherapy Effectiveness

- Its bioactive compounds like aloin and aloe-emodin, enhance the effects of chemotherapy by inhibiting cancer cell growth and inducing apoptosis.

- It protects healthy cells from radiation damage and makes cancer cells more sensitive to radiotherapy.

- Directly inhibits cancer cell growth, slowing tumor progression.

Protection against Treatment Toxicity

It neutralizes oxidative stress caused by chemotherapy and radiotherapy, reducing side effects like inflammation and tissue damage. It supports liver and kidney function by promoting toxin elimination.

Reduction of Treatment Side Effects

- It soothes the gastrointestinal tract, alleviating chemotherapy-induced nausea, vomiting, and digestive disturbances.

- It helps heal mucous membranes, reducing the severity of mucositis.

- It Promotes faster healing of radiation-induced burns.

Immune System Support

- It boosts immune function by enhancing macrophages, T-cells, and NK cells, which are crucial for targeting cancer cells.

- It helps prevent infections during treatment.

Anti-Inflammatory and Pain Relief

- It reduces chronic inflammation and alleviates joint and muscle pain during treatment.

- It helps reduce cancer-related pain, potentially reducing the need for strong painkillers.

Improvement in Quality of Life

- Boosts energy levels and reduces fatigue.

- Improves gut health, ensuring better nutrient absorption.

- Reduces anxiety and depression by alleviating physical symptoms.

Direct Anti-Cancer Properties

- Directly induces cancer cell death without harming healthy tissue.

- Inhibits the formation of new blood vessels to tumors, starving and slowing their growth.

Recovery and Healing

- Supports immune function, reduces inflammation, and promotes faster healing.

- Improves mental health and emotional resilience during the cancer journey.

Clinical Studies and Testimonials

Clinical studies have shown that Aloe arborescens can provide significant benefits for cancer patients, both in enhancing immune response and improving quality of life. A study published in the Journal of Cancer Research and Clinical Oncology found that Aloe arborescens extract, when used alongside chemotherapy, helped reduce the toxic side effects of the treatment while enhancing its effectiveness. The extract appeared to protect healthy cells from chemotherapy-induced damage and helped in reducing fatigue and other common side effects.

A clinical trial conducted by the National Center for Biotechnology Information (NCBI) demonstrated that Aloe arborescens extract helped improve immune function by increasing the activity of natural killer (NK) cells and T-lymphocytes, which are crucial for the body's ability to fight cancer. Patients using Aloe arborescens alongside their conventional treatments reported improved energy levels, better tolerance to chemotherapy, and an enhanced sense of well-being.

In "Cancer can be cured," the author recited how a lot of people had their cancer cured by using a Brazilian recipe of Aloe Arborescens juice with honey and some distillate. The types of cancer cured had a wide range from prostate to head and neck cancers. In the introduction, I also mentioned how Thora's father lived cancer-free for over 15 years until passing away after using this recipe alongside conventional treatment. The following youtube video shows how to make this mix: https://youtu.be/iZtBLFNbhJY?si=r6HyqqAF3qJ8pIYr

Patient Testimonials: Cancer patients who have used Aloe arborescens as part of their treatment plan reported positive outcomes, such as reduced nausea, improved digestion, and faster recovery times. Some patients have noted that applying the gel helped alleviate radiation burns and skin irritation while consuming aloe juice supported their immune function and overall vitality. Many have found Aloe arborescens a gentle yet effective addition to their cancer treatment, providing both physical relief and emotional support during a challenging time.

Practical Applications

Aloe juice can be consumed or used topically to soothe burns and support digestion. It can also be added to smoothies or taken in supplement form. A common recipe for fighting cancer alone or alongside standard treatment is to mix the juice of two aloe arborescens leaves (aged over five years) with half a kilo of raw honey and 2-3 tablespoons of distilled liquor, such as whiskey, tequila, vodka, or cognac.

Bitter Melon

Bitter melon (Momordica charantia), native to Asia and Africa, is used in traditional medicine for blood sugar regulation and digestive health. Recent research suggests it has anti-cancer properties due to compounds like charantin and momordicoside, which may induce apoptosis, inhibit cancer cell proliferation, and regulate blood sugar.

How Bitter Melon May Help Fight Cancer

- Bitter melon extract can trigger apoptosis in cancer cells, helping reduce tumor growth.

- It inhibits the growth of cancer cells by targeting key pathways like mTOR and AMPK, which are involved in cancer cell metabolism and growth through cancer stem cells.

- Its Anti-inflammatory and antioxidant properties may help reduce chemotherapy side effects Bitter melon has antioxidants that protect healthy cells but may interfere with treatments relying on oxidative stress.

- It helps lower blood sugar, benefiting cancers linked to insulin resistance, such as breast and pancreatic cancers.

Types of Cancer Bitter Melon May Help

Bitter melon is beneficial for breast, pancreatic, colon, liver, prostate, gastric, leukemia, and skin cancers.

Breast Cancer: Inhibits cell proliferation through pathways like mTOR.

Pancreatic Cancer: Induces apoptosis and increases sensitivity of cancer stem cells to chemotherapy.

Colon Cancer: Inhibits growth through apoptosis and inflammation regulation.

Lung and Prostate Cancer: Reduces proliferation and modulates pathways involved in cell survival.

Clinical Studies

Studies show bitter melon can induce apoptosis and inhibit cancer growth. It has immune-boosting effects, enhancing NK cell activity. Patients report improved chemotherapy tolerance, reduced fatigue, and better immune function.

Patient Testimonials: Patients have noted benefits like reduced fatigue, better digestion, and improved energy. Bitter melon also helped regulate blood sugar, supporting those at risk of hyperglycemia.

Black Cumin

Black cumin seeds (Nigella sativa), known for their healing properties across the Middle East and Asia, have potential benefits in cancer treatment. The active compound thymoquinone shows promise in enhancing chemotherapy, protecting against its side effects, and improving patients' quality of life for several types of cancer, including breast, colon, prostate, lung, pancreatic and liver cancers.

How Black Cumin Supports Cancer Therapy

Enhancement of Chemotherapy Effectiveness

- Black cumin, particularly thymoquinone, increases cancer cells' sensitivity to treatment.

- Promotes cancer cell death, enhancing chemotherapy's anti-tumor effects.

- Slows cancer cell proliferation and metastasis.

- Protects Against Chemotherapy Toxicity

- Reduces oxidative stress and protects healthy cells from chemotherapy-induced damage.

- Preserves liver, kidney, and heart function during chemotherapy.

Reduction of Chemotherapy Side Effects

- Alleviates nausea, vomiting, and digestive discomfort.

- Boosts immune function, reducing vulnerability to infections.

Anti-Inflammatory Effects

- Helps alleviate chronic inflammation, improving well-being.

Improvement in Quality of Life

- Provides analgesic effects, reducing cancer-related pain.

- Reduces fatigue and improves vitality.

- Supports mood and reduces anxiety and depression.

Overcoming Drug Resistance

- Thymoquinone may help reverse drug resistance, enhancing the long-term effectiveness of chemotherapy.

Support for Detoxification

- Protects liver function, aiding in the detoxification of chemotherapy drugs.

Direct Anti-Cancer Activity

- Thymoquinone inhibits cancer cell proliferation and promotes cell death, making black cumin a promising complementary therapy.

Clinical Studies

Clinical studies have shown that black cumin seeds can significantly benefit cancer patients, particularly in boosting immunity and reducing tumor growth. A study published in the Journal of Cancer Research and Therapeutics demonstrated that black cumin seed extract could inhibit cancer cell proliferation and reduce tumor size.

A clinical trial conducted by the National Center for Biotechnology Information (NCBI) demonstrated that black cumin seed oil helped improve immune function in cancer patients by increasing the activity of natural killer (NK) cells and other immune components. Patients who used black cumin seed oil as part of their treatment plan reported better energy levels, reduced fatigue, and improved overall well-being.

A 2010 preclinical study reported in suggests that administration of NSO or TQ can lower cyclophosphamide (CTX) induced toxicity, as shown by an up-regulation of antioxidant mechanisms.

Evidence from preclinical studies reported in 2017 indicated that thymoquinone in black cumin can increase the effectiveness of conventional cancer treatments while protecting normal cells from therapy-associated toxic effects.

A retrospective clinical study reported in with 20 patients who had non-metastatic locally advanced inoperable pancreatic cancer revealed that consumption of black cumin oil and pure honey before and during chemoradiotherapy increased their survival time by 50%.

A study reported in Digestive Diseases and Science, 2015, found that consumption of black cumin containing thymoquinone before and following *gemcitabine* treatment caused increased apoptosis in *pancreatic* cancer cells and inhibited tumor growth.

Patient Testimonials: Cancer patients who have incorporated black cumin seeds into their diet or treatment plan reported positive outcomes, such as reduced inflammation, improved immune function, and better tolerance to conventional treatments. Many patients have found that using black cumin oil in cooking or taking it as a supplement helped alleviate side effects like joint pain and digestive discomfort while also providing an energy boost. Testimonials also highlight the versatility of black cumin, with patients using it in both culinary and supplemental forms to support their overall health during cancer treatment.

Blueberries

Blueberries have been used for centuries across various cultures for their health-promoting properties. Traditionally, Indigenous populations in North America valued blueberries not only as a nutritious food source but also for medicinal purposes.

Potential Benefits of Blueberries in Cancer Treatment

Antioxidant Properties: Blueberries are rich in antioxidants, which help neutralize free radicals, reducing oxidative stress that can contribute to cancer development.

Anti-inflammatory Effects: Chronic inflammation is associated with cancer progression. Blueberries contain compounds like quercetin and resveratrol that may help reduce inflammation.

Apoptosis and Cell Cycle Regulation: Blueberry polyphenols may encourage apoptosis (programmed cell death) in cancer cells and slow their proliferation, particularly in breast, colon, and prostate cancers.

Anti-metastatic Effects: Some compounds in blueberries can inhibit enzymes and signaling pathways involved in metastasis, potentially reducing cancer spread.

Chemotherapy Support: Blueberries may enhance the effects of chemotherapy. For example, they have been studied for their potential to improve response to treatments like doxorubicin in breast cancer.

Flaxseeds

Flax seeds (Linum usitatissimum), cultivated for thousands of years, are rich in omega-3 fatty acids, lignans, and fiber, which provide multiple benefits in cancer treatment and prevention. They enhance standard therapies, reduce side effects, and improve quality of life for cancer patients.

How Flaxseeds Help in Cancer Care

Enhancement of Treatment Effectiveness

Inhibition of Hormone-Related Cancers: Lignans in flax seeds inhibit hormone-related cancers, such as breast and prostate, by reducing active estrogen levels.

Tumor Growth Inhibition: Omega-3s and lignans block cancer cell proliferation and induce apoptosis.

Anti-Angiogenesis: Flax seeds prevent the formation of new blood vessels for tumors, starving cancer cells of nutrients.

Protection against Treatment Toxicity

Cell Protection: Omega-3s protect healthy cells from chemotherapy and radiotherapy damage.

Antioxidant Support: Lignans and omega-3s help neutralize free radicals, reducing organ toxicity and side effects like fatigue.

Reduction of Treatment Side Effects

Gastrointestinal Support: Fiber in flax seeds alleviates constipation and nausea, improving digestive health.

Inflammation Reduction: Omega-3s reduce inflammation, easing mucositis and skin irritation.

Fatigue Reduction: Omega-3s combat chemotherapy-induced fatigue, enhancing energy.

Immune System Support

Immune Modulation: Lignans and omega-3s enhance immune function, helping the body recover during treatment.

Antimicrobial Properties: Bioactive compounds help protect against infections.

Hormonal Regulation

Hormone-Dependent Cancers: Lignans help regulate estrogen, slowing hormone-driven tumor growth.

Anti-Inflammatory Effects

Systemic Inflammation Reduction: Omega-3s reduce inflammation, alleviating pain and discomfort.

Pain Relief: Reduces joint and muscle pain associated with chemotherapy.

Heart and Vascular Protection

Cardioprotective Properties: Omega-3s protect the heart from chemotherapy-induced damage.

Blood Health Support: Nutrients support healthy blood production, reducing anemia.

Improvement in Quality of Life

Mood and Cognitive Support: Omega-3s protect brain function, reducing cognitive issues and improving mood.

Enhanced Energy: Antioxidants and omega-3s boost energy levels, reducing fatigue.

Direct Anti-Cancer Properties

Apoptosis Induction: Promotes cancer cell death, particularly in hormone-related cancers.

Anti-Metastatic Effects: Reduces cancer spread by inhibiting angiogenesis and inflammation.

Support for Detoxification

Liver Health: Nutrients support liver detoxification, reducing chemotherapy-induced damage.

Improved Toxin Elimination: Fiber aids in toxin elimination, reducing the burden on detoxifying organs.

Clinical Studies and Patient Testimonials

Clinical studies indicate that flaxseeds can slow tumor growth, modulate hormone levels, and improve prognosis in hormone-related cancers, such as breast and prostate cancers. Patients report reduced fatigue, improved digestion, and better overall well-being by adding flaxseeds to their diets.

Fucoidan

Fucoidan, derived from brown seaweeds like wakame and kombu, has been traditionally used in Japan and Korea for wellness and longevity. It is now gaining attention for its potential benefits in cancer treatment, including anticancer, anti-inflammatory, and immune-boosting properties. Fucoidan is available in extract capsules. But the quality varies with suppliers.

How Fucoidan Helps Cancer Patients

Anticancer Properties: Fucoidan induces apoptosis (cancer cell death) and inhibits angiogenesis, which restricts tumor growth by starving cancer cells of nutrients.

Immune System Support: Fucoidan boosts immune cell activity, enhancing the body's ability to target and eliminate cancer cells, especially during treatment that weakens immunity.

Reducing Chemotherapy Side Effects: Fucoidan helps protect healthy cells and alleviate side effects such as nausea and immune suppression, making chemotherapy more tolerable.

Inhibition of Metastasis: Fucoidan interferes with cancer cell adhesion and migration, preventing metastasis.

Anti-Inflammatory Effects: It reduces chronic inflammation, supporting overall health during cancer treatment.

Clinical Evidence

Preclinical Studies: Fucoidan has been shown to inhibit the growth of various cancers and enhance chemotherapy's effectiveness.

Clinical Trials: Fucoidan supplementation improved quality of life, reduced fatigue, and enhanced immune function in cancer patients.

Patient Testimonials: Users report improved energy levels, reduced side effects, and overall better well-being.

Garlic

Garlic (Allium sativum) has been used in traditional medicine for its antibacterial, antiviral, and antifungal properties. It supports heart health, enhances immunity, and has potential benefits in cancer prevention and treatment.

Benefits of Garlic for Cancer Patients

Immune System Support: Garlic boosts immune function, enhancing natural killer (NK) cell activity, which is crucial for targeting cancer cells.

Anticancer Properties: Sulfur compounds like allicin and DADS promote apoptosis, inhibit cancer cell growth, and reduce the risk of cancers like colorectal, stomach, and prostate.

Antioxidant and Anti-inflammatory Effects: Rich in antioxidants, garlic fights oxidative stress and inflammation, which can drive cancer progression. It also inhibits cancer cell proliferation.

Cardiovascular Benefits: Garlic helps reduce blood pressure and cholesterol, supporting cardiovascular health, particularly in patients undergoing treatment.

Detoxification and Chemoprotection: Garlic aids detoxification, potentially reducing the toxic effects of chemotherapy by enhancing liver enzyme activity.

Patient Testimonials

Cancer patients using garlic report improved immunity and overall health during treatment, making it a useful complementary therapy.

Ginger

Ginger (*Zingiber officinale*) has been used in traditional medicine for thousands of years for its anti-inflammatory, digestive, and warming properties. It is now being studied for its potential benefits in cancer treatment.

Benefits of Ginger for Cancer Patients

Nausea and Vomiting Reduction: Ginger effectively reduces chemotherapy-induced nausea and vomiting (CINV). Studies have shown significant reductions in nausea severity in patients who took ginger during chemotherapy.

Anti-Inflammatory and Antioxidant Effects: Ginger contains compounds like gingerol and shogaol, which reduce chronic inflammation and oxidative stress. This may help lower cancer risk and progression.

Pain Relief: Ginger helps alleviate joint pain caused by cancer treatments, such as those involving hormone-sensitive breast cancer.

Appetite Stimulation and Improved Digestion: Ginger aids digestion and appetite, helping cancer patients maintain adequate nutrition during treatment.

Anticancer Properties (Preclinical Evidence): Compounds in ginger have been found to inhibit cancer cell growth and promote apoptosis in various types of cancer in preclinical studies.

Patient Testimonials

Patients using ginger report better tolerance of chemotherapy, improved appetite, and relief from nausea and digestive issues, contributing to an enhanced quality of life.

Honey

Honey has been used for centuries for its antibacterial, anti-inflammatory, and wound-healing properties. It has potential as a complementary therapy for various cancers due to its rich antioxidant and anti-inflammatory properties.

Benefits of Honey for Cancer Patients

Enhancement of Chemotherapy: Honey's phenolic compounds can enhance chemotherapy effectiveness by increasing cancer cell sensitivity, inhibiting tumor growth, and preventing metastasis.

Protection against Chemotherapy Toxicity: Honey helps protect organs like the liver and kidneys from chemotherapy damage through its antioxidant properties.

Reduction of Chemotherapy Side Effects: Honey reduces oral mucositis, gastrointestinal issues like nausea, and chemotherapy-induced fatigue, thanks to its soothing and anti-inflammatory effects.

Immune System Support: Honey boosts immune function and helps prevent infections in immunocompromised patients.

Anti-Inflammatory and Pain Management: Honey reduces systemic inflammation, alleviating pain and swelling, and has natural pain-relieving properties.

Mood and Mental Health Support: Honey's antioxidants help reduce anxiety and depression and may provide cognitive support during treatment.

Improvement in Quality of Life: Honey helps boost energy levels, improve appetite, and promote better sleep, enhancing overall well-being during treatment.

Direct Anticancer Effects: Honey exhibits anti-tumor properties, including inhibiting cancer cell growth and promoting apoptosis.

Clinical Studies

Clinical studies have shown that Honey, particularly Manuka honey, can benefit cancer patients significantly. A study published in the Journal of Clinical Oncology found that Manuka honey can reduce the severity of oral mucositis, a painful condition often experienced by patients undergoing chemotherapy and radiation therapy. The antibacterial and anti-inflammatory properties of honey help promote wound healing and reduce inflammation, making it a valuable complementary therapy.

A clinical trial conducted by the National Center for Biotechnology Information (NCBI) demonstrated that Honey can improve the quality of life for cancer patients by reducing symptoms like sore throat, gastrointestinal discomfort, and fatigue. The study highlighted Honey's role in supporting immune health, which is crucial for patients undergoing treatments that weaken their immune systems.

Patient Testimonials: Cancer patients who have used Honey as part of their treatment reported positive outcomes, such as reduced mouth sores, improved digestion, and better overall well-being. Many patients have found that taking a spoonful of Manuka honey daily helped soothe their throat and reduce radiation-induced skin irritation. Testimonials also highlight the use of Honey in teas or smoothies as a natural way to support energy levels and enhance immune function during treatment.

Mistletoe

Mistletoe (Viscum album) has been used in complementary cancer therapies, particularly in Europe, for its immune-boosting and anticancer properties. It is often administered as liquid extract via subcutaneous injections to enhance patients' quality of life during cancer treatment.

Benefits of Mistletoe for Cancer Patients

Immune System Modulation: Mistletoe extract stimulates the immune system by increasing the activity of immune cells like NK cells and T-lymphocytes, helping the body target cancer cells more effectively.

Inducing Apoptosis: Compounds in mistletoe, such as viscotoxins and lectins, induce apoptosis in cancer cells without harming healthy cells, limiting tumor growth.

Reducing Chemotherapy Side Effects: Mistletoe helps reduce chemotherapy side effects like fatigue, nausea, and pain, making treatments more manageable.

Anti-Inflammatory Effects: Mistletoe reduces chronic inflammation, which can aid overall well-being in cancer patients.

Improving Quality of Life: Mistletoe therapy boosts energy, reduces pain, and supports emotional health, helping with anxiety and depression.

Clinical Evidence

Studies: Research shows mistletoe can induce apoptosis in cancer cells and improve quality of life for patients undergoing chemotherapy.

Trials: Randomized trials indicate mistletoe can enhance survival rates and reduce the need for pain medication in advanced cancer patients.

Patient Testimonials: Many patients report reduced treatment side effects, improved energy, and overall better quality of life.

Papaya Leaves and Seeds

Papaya leaves and seeds, traditionally used in Central America, have antibacterial, anti-inflammatory, and digestive benefits. They are now being studied for their anticancer properties, showing promise in enhancing chemotherapy and radiotherapy for various cancers, including breast, liver, lung, and prostate.

Benefits of Papaya Leaves and Seeds for Cancer Patients

Anticancer Properties: Papaya leaves and seeds contain compounds like acetogenins and flavonoids that induce apoptosis, inhibit cancer cell growth, and prevent angiogenesis, effectively starving tumors.

Enhancement of Chemotherapy and Radiotherapy: Bioactive compounds, such as flavonoids and papain, increase chemotherapy efficacy while protecting healthy cells from damage, improving treatment outcomes.

Reduction of Side Effects: Papaya leaves help boost immune function, protect platelets, and reduce nausea and digestive issues caused by treatment. Vitamins B and C help reduce fatigue and improve energy levels.

Antioxidant and Anti-Inflammatory Effects: Rich in antioxidants, papaya leaves reduce oxidative stress and inflammation, protecting healthy tissues and reducing discomfort.

Detoxification Support: Papaya seeds support liver and kidney health, enhancing detoxification and reducing organ damage during chemotherapy.

Immune System Modulation: Papaya leaves stimulate immune cells, boosting defenses against infections during treatment.

Hormonal Balance: Compounds in papaya seeds help regulate hormone levels, potentially benefiting hormone-sensitive cancers like breast and prostate.

Improvement in Quality of Life: Nutrients in papaya leaves reduce fatigue and pain, improving overall energy and comfort for cancer patients.

Cancer Prevention: Papaya compounds may act preventively by protecting against DNA damage and oxidative stress that contribute to cancer.

Mental and Emotional Well-Being: Antioxidant properties may help protect against cognitive decline and improve emotional health during treatment.

Clinical Evidence

Studies have shown that papaya leaf extract can improve platelet counts and immune function in cancer patients. Compounds in papaya seeds also exhibit anticancer effects, promoting apoptosis and inhibiting cell growth.

Patient Testimonials: Cancer patients who have used papaya leaves, fruit, and seeds as part of their treatment plan reported improved overall well-being, better digestion, and enhanced immune function. Many patients have found that consuming papaya leaf juice helped boost their platelet counts and reduced chemotherapy-induced fatigue. The seeds have improved digestion and support liver health when consumed in small amounts. At the same time, the fruit has helped alleviate gastrointestinal discomfort and provided essential nutrients supporting their recovery.

Perilla Leaves and Seed Oil

Perilla (Perilla frutescens), used in traditional East Asian medicine, is rich in bioactive compounds like omega-3 fatty acids, flavonoids, and polyphenols. It shows potential as a complementary therapy in cancer treatment.

Key Benefits of Perilla for Cancer Patients

Anticancer Properties: Compounds like rosmarinic acid and luteolin induce apoptosis, inhibit cancer cell proliferation, and prevent angiogenesis, helping limit tumor growth.

Enhancement of Chemotherapy and Radiotherapy: Omega-3s and flavonoids increase cancer cells' sensitivity to chemotherapy and protect healthy cells, reducing side effects.

Reduction of Treatment Side Effects: Perilla helps alleviate nausea, fatigue, and inflammation caused by cancer treatments.

Antioxidant Support: Rich in antioxidants, perilla neutralizes free radicals and protects cells from oxidative stress.

Immune System Support: Perilla modulates immune response, boosts white blood cell count, and helps prevent infections during treatment.

Anti-Metastatic Properties: Alpha-linolenic acid (ALA) inhibits cancer metastasis and targets cancer stem cells, reducing the risk of relapse.

Liver Protection and Detoxification: Perilla supports liver health, aiding detoxification and protecting against chemotherapy-induced damage.

Cardiovascular Protection: Omega-3s in perilla support heart health and reduce the risk of cardiotoxicity from cancer treatments.

Improvement in Quality of Life: Omega-3s and essential oils reduce stress, improve mood, and help with cognitive issues related to treatment.

Hormonal Regulation: Phytoestrogens in perilla help modulate hormone levels, beneficial for hormone-sensitive cancers like breast and prostate.

Skin Health Support: Perilla's anti-inflammatory properties protect against radiation dermatitis and promote skin repair.

Clinical Evidence

Studies show that perilla reduces inflammation, boosts immunity, and improves cardiovascular health. Patients using perilla report reduced fatigue, improved well-being, and better management of treatment side effects.

Probiotics and Fermented Foods

Fermented foods like kimchi, sauerkraut, and yogurt have been used worldwide for digestive health and immune support. Probiotics and fermented foods are gaining attention for their potential benefits in cancer care, particularly in supporting gut health, boosting immunity, and reducing treatment side effects.

Benefits of Probiotics for Cancer Patients

Improved Gut Health: Probiotics help restore a healthy gut microbiome disrupted by chemotherapy and radiotherapy, reducing gastrointestinal issues like diarrhea, constipation, and nausea.

Immune System Support: Probiotics modulate immune responses, boosting immune cells like macrophages and NK cells, which help target cancer cells.

Reduction of Inflammation: Probiotics help reduce systemic inflammation by regulating cytokine levels, supporting overall health during treatment.

Enhanced Nutrient Absorption: Probiotics support gut health, improving nutrient absorption and preventing malnutrition during cancer treatment.

Prevention of Infections: Probiotics help maintain a healthy balance of gut bacteria, reducing the risk of infections in immunocompromised patients.

Reduced Cancer Therapy Side Effects: Probiotics reduce side effects like mucositis, fatigue, and dermatitis caused by chemotherapy and radiation.

Potential Anticancer Properties: Some probiotics produce metabolites that may inhibit cancer cell growth and enhance immune responses.

Benefits of Fermented Foods

Fermented foods such as kefir, miso, and kombucha contain probiotics and bioactive compounds that support digestion, immune health, and reduce inflammation. Regular consumption of fermented dairy has been linked to a reduced risk of colorectal cancer.

Turmeric

Turmeric, used in traditional medicine for centuries, contains curcumin, which has potential benefits for cancer patients by enhancing conventional treatments and reducing side effects.

Key Benefits for Cancer Patients

Enhancing Effectiveness of Cancer Therapies: Curcumin inhibits cancer-promoting pathways (e.g., NF-κB, STAT3), enhances chemotherapy and radiotherapy effectiveness, and makes cancer cells more sensitive to treatment by inhibiting drug resistance.

Reducing Adverse Effects: Curcumin's antioxidant and anti-inflammatory properties protect healthy cells from damage caused by chemotherapy and radiotherapy, mitigating side effects like fatigue, nausea, and organ toxicity.

Immune System Support: Curcumin boosts immune function, enhancing the activity of immune cells like NK cells and T-cells to help the body target cancer more effectively.

Chronic Inflammation Reduction: By reducing inflammation, curcumin can make tumors more vulnerable to treatment and slow cancer progression.

Potential Synergy with Other Drugs: Curcumin works well with certain chemotherapy drugs, enhancing their effects while reducing side effects.

Clinical Evidence

Studies show that curcumin can reduce tumor growth, increase chemotherapy effectiveness, and minimize treatment toxicity. Patients report reduced side effects like joint pain, nausea, and fatigue, leading to improved quality of life.

Virgin Coconut Oil (VCO)

Virgin coconut oil, traditionally used in tropical regions, has gained attention for its potential role in supporting cancer therapies. Rich in medium-chain fatty acids (MCFAs), antioxidants, and bioactive compounds, it may enhance treatment effectiveness and reduce side effects.

Key Benefits for Cancer Patients

Enhancing Treatment Effectiveness : Antioxidants in VCO help protect healthy cells and make cancer cells more vulnerable to chemotherapy.

Boosting Energy: MCFAs provide energy to healthy cells, helping them maintain function during chemotherapy.

Antitumor Effects: Lauric acid induces apoptosis and inhibits cancer cell growth, potentially reducing tumors.

Chemotherapy Sensitivity: Antioxidants in VCO help protect healthy cells and make cancer cells more vulnerable to chemotherapy.

Reducing Side Effects of Treatment

Inflammation and Oxidative Stress: VCO's antioxidants reduce inflammation and oxidative damage, protecting against side effects like mucositis and skin irritation.

Organ Protection: VCO supports liver, kidney, and heart health, reducing chemotherapy-induced toxicity.

Digestive Health: VCO alleviates digestive issues, such as nausea and vomiting, by reducing inflammation and improving gut health.

Immune System Support

Boosting Immunity: Lauric acid has antimicrobial properties, supporting immune function during treatment.

Immune Modulation: VCO modulates immune responses, reducing chronic inflammation while enhancing defense mechanisms.

Nutritional Support and Quality of Life

Energy and Nutrient Absorption: VCO is calorie-dense and supports absorption of fat-soluble vitamins, improving overall energy and nutritional status.

Skin Health: VCO soothes radiation dermatitis, reducing dryness and irritation.

Potential Synergy with Ketogenic Diets

Metabolic Therapy: VCO supports ketosis, which may deprive cancer cells of glucose while providing energy to healthy cells.

Cognitive Support: MCFAs provide alternative energy for the brain, potentially improving cognitive function during chemotherapy.

Clinical Evidence

Studies show VCO supports immune health, protects organs, and reduces chemotherapy side effects like fatigue and nausea. Patients report improved energy, better digestion, and enhanced well-being.

Patient Testimonials: Cancer patients who have incorporated virgin coconut oil into their treatment regimen reported improvements in energy levels, reduced gastrointestinal discomfort, and better overall well-being. For instance, some patients have found that adding coconut oil to their diet helped alleviate the dryness and irritation caused by radiation therapy. In contrast, others noted improved digestion and fewer issues with chemotherapy-induced nausea.

Julie Figueroa, a former computer company executive, was diagnosed with aggressive breast cancer in 1998 despite receiving a clean bill of health earlier that year. After undergoing surgery and chemotherapy, the cancer persisted and later spread to her skull in 2001. Following another surgery, her prognosis remained grim. The cancer was so close to the brain's main artery that twenty percent of it remained there. Julie returned to her farm in the Philippines, where she explored medicinal plants to strengthen her immune system. She came across research on coconut oil and began consuming it regularly. After six months, her cancer went into remission, which she attributes to the use of virgin coconut oil, leading to her being cancer-free today.

Conclusion

This chapter raises the need of conventional cancer treatments for complementary help to increase their effectiveness and avoid their adverse effects on the patients' general well-being and quality of life. It has shown that there are 15 common products, which, when included in the treatment plan, can help increase the treatment outcomes and maintain a desired quality of life for patients. However, these natural therapies may have adverse interactions and may even negatively affect the effectiveness of some specific chemotherapy and immunotherapy drugs. The next chapter will guide you which drugs and which natural products should not be used alongside each other.

Chapter 6

Navigating Potential Risks - Avoiding Harmful Interactions

Stay safe and informed—know what to watch for when combining therapies.

When exploring the benefits of plant-based therapies in cancer treatment, it is essential to remain aware of potential risks and interactions. Some natural products may interfere with conventional cancer drugs, reducing effectiveness or even increasing harmful side effects. By understanding these risks, we can make informed choices that enhance our health while avoiding unintended consequences.

This chapter will discuss unwanted interactions between plant-based therapies and conventional cancer treatments, providing practical guidance on avoiding these adverse effects. We will also explore how to work with healthcare providers to ensure a safe, integrated approach to cancer care. The goal is to help you make the most of natural and conventional treatments without compromising safety or effectiveness.

Avoiding Unwanted Interactions

Certain natural products may interact with chemotherapy, targeted therapy, immunotherapy, or hormonal therapy drugs, potentially affecting their effectiveness or causing side effects. For example, plant-based products like Aloe arborescens, bitter melon, black cumin, turmeric, and virgin coconut oil may interfere with cancer treatments by enhancing or reducing their potency. Each product has specific properties that can either support or hinder cancer treatment—depending on the drug or therapy.

It is essential to understand these potential interactions to make safe decisions about combining natural and conventional therapies.

Practical Guidance for Safety

Careful planning and open communication with healthcare providers is the best way to avoid negative interactions. Here are some general guidelines to ensure safety:

Consult Your Healthcare Provider: Before adding any herbal remedy or supplement to your treatment plan, talk to your oncologist. They can help you understand potential risks and adjust your treatment regimen.

Timing and Dosage: When taking natural products and prescribed medications, be mindful of timing and dosage. Spacing out the timing of doses or adjusting the amount taken can avoid some interactions.

Avoid Self-Medication: Even if a natural product is widely regarded as beneficial, avoid self-medication without consulting your healthcare team. Many herbs and supplements have complex effects that could lead to unintended consequences if not carefully monitored.

3. Consulting Your Healthcare Team

Effective communication with our healthcare team is crucial to safely integrating natural therapies into our cancer care. Here are some tips on how to approach this:

Prepare Information: When discussing natural products, be ready to provide information about what we plan to take, including its intended benefits, how we plan to take it, and where we sourced it.

Ask Questions: Do not hesitate to ask your healthcare provider about potential interactions and how best to avoid them. It is also helpful to ask whether laboratory tests are needed to monitor possible interactions.

Document Everything: Record all anti-cancer foods /spices and supplements you take. This way can help your healthcare team track what might influence your treatment outcomes.

Common Unwanted Interactions listed by natural products

For each specific plant-based product and supplement, we can identify cancer drugs that may have unwanted interactions, explain why they may occur, and suggest ways to minimize adverse effects.

Aloe Arborescens:

- Aloe arborescens is known to interact with several chemotherapy drugs, including *doxorubicin, cisplatin, cyclophosphamide, and 5-Fluorouracil (5-FU)*.

- The antioxidant properties of aloe can interfere with these drugs, potentially reducing their effectiveness by counteracting the oxidative stress mechanism that some chemotherapy agents rely on.

- Aloe also has gastrointestinal effects that may alter the absorption of these drugs, impacting their efficacy.

- If we must take the above drugs or immunotherapy drugs, we can minimize adverse interactions by limiting daily intake to ¼ cups of juice at least 2 hours after taking medication. We should also discuss using aloe arborescens during treatment with our healthcare provider.

Bitter Melon:

- Bitter melon is rich in antioxidants, which may interfere with the effectiveness of chemotherapy drugs like *cisplatin and doxorubicin*.

- These drugs depend on oxidative stress to target and kill cancer cells, and the antioxidant activity of bitter melon may reduce their impact. Additionally, bitter melon affects blood sugar levels, which could lead to complications if used with diabetes medications.

- If we must take the above drugs or diabetes medications, we should avoid bitter melon without medical supervision, as it may alter treatment outcomes and glucose control. With medical supervision, we can minimize the interactions by using low doses, e.g., a small portion of juice or a few capsules 1-2 hours after taking medication.

Black Cumin:

- Black cumin contains thymoquinone, which can interfere with liver enzymes responsible for metabolizing chemotherapy drugs such as ***cyclophosphamide, doxorubicin, and paclitaxel.***

- This interaction may lead to altered drug concentrations in the body, reducing effectiveness or increasing toxicity. Thymoquinone can modulate the cytochrome P450 enzyme system in the liver, which is critical for processing many chemotherapy agents.

- To minimize the adverse interactions if you must take the above drugs, you should take ½ to 1 tsp per day of black seed oil or black seeds at least from 1-2 hours of taking medication. You should also inform and discuss with your healthcare provider.

Blueberries:

- Blueberries, especially in concentrated forms like extracts, can interact with certain cancer drugs. These interactions are often due to blueberries' effects on enzymes that metabolize drugs, primarily cytochrome P450 enzymes, which can lead to either reduced effectiveness or increased toxicity of medications. Here are some examples of drugs and suggestions to minimize interactions: *Tamoxifen, Irinotecan, Erlotinib (Tarceva), Cyclophosphamide, Bortezomib (Velcade),*

- To reduce the risk of unwanted interactions, we should eat small servings (1/2 cup per day) of whole blueberries rather than extracts or concentrated forms and separate the intake of blueberries from medication times by 1-2 hours, especially with drugs that rely on stomach acidity for absorption.

Flax Seeds:

- Flax seeds are rich in lignans and omega-3 fatty acids, which can affect hormone levels and interact with hormone-based cancer treatments, such as *tamoxifen and letrozole*. Flax seeds also have blood-thinning properties, which may increase the risk of bleeding when used with anticoagulants like *warfarin*.

- It is best to have the above drugs replaced with other medications. But if we must take them, we should limit our intake of flaxseeds to 1 tablespoon per day at least 1-2 hours apart from cancer medication to minimize adverse interactions with them. It is also essential to discuss incorporating flax seeds into our diet with our oncologist.

Fucoidan:

- Fucoidan, derived from brown seaweed, is known for its anti-cancer properties but can interact with chemotherapy drugs, such as *cisplatin, doxorubicin, and cyclophosphamide*, and anticoagulants like *warfarin and heparin* by altering immune function and increasing bleeding risk. Fucoidan may also affect how certain chemotherapy drugs are metabolized, leading to either reduced efficacy or increased toxicity.

- To minimize adverse interactions with chemo drugs, we should take fucoidan with food at least 1-2 hours after taking medication. We should also discuss this with our healthcare provider before using fucoidan to determine the safety of combining it with their treatment.

Garlic:

- Garlic has potent antioxidant properties that can interfere with chemotherapy drugs that rely on oxidative stress to kill cancer cells, such as *cyclophosphamide, doxorubicin, and cisplatin*. Garlic may also affect blood clotting and interact with anticoagulants like warfarin and aspirin, increasing the risk of bleeding.

- Suppose we must undergo chemotherapy with the above drugs or take blood thinners. In that case, we should use 1-2 cloves of garlic daily at least 2 hours apart from medication and avoid to minimize adverse interactions. It is important to discuss our garlic use openly with our oncologist.

Ginger:

- Ginger is known for its anti-nausea and anti-inflammatory properties. Still, it may interact with blood-thinning medications, such as ***warfarin and aspirin***, and chemotherapy drugs, like ***cyclophosphamide and doxorubicin***, by enhancing their effects. This effect can lead to increased bleeding risk or altered drug metabolism.

- It is best not to take these drugs. But if we must, we should limit our intake to no more than one teaspoon of fresh or dried ginger per day and at least 1 hour apart from medication to minimize adverse interactions. It is important to discuss ginger supplements openly with our healthcare provider before using them.

Honey:

- Honey, particularly Manuka honey, has antibacterial and immune-modulating properties that can interact with immunotherapy drugs, such as *pembrolizumab, nivolumab, and ipilimumab*, by enhancing immune system activity. This interaction may lead to an overactive immune response, potentially causing adverse effects.

- If we must take the above drugs, we can minimize their adverse interaction with honey by taking 1-2 teaspoons daily with food separately for at least 1-2 hours from medication. However, it is always important to consult our healthcare provider before using honey, especially during immunotherapy.

Papaya:

- Papaya leaves, fruit, and seeds contain enzymes and compounds that may interact with chemotherapy drugs that rely on liver enzymes for metabolization and absorption, such as ***cyclophosphamide and doxorubicin***, potentially altering their efficacy.

- To minimize adverse interactions with these drugs, we should sparingly use papaya leaves and seeds and avoid them within 1-2 hours of chemotherapy. It is important to consult our healthcare provider before using papaya products to determine their safety alongside treatment.

Perilla:

- Perilla leaves and seed oil contain rosmarinic acid, which has anti-inflammatory effects. Still, it can also interact with liver-metabolized drugs, such as specific chemotherapy and targeted therapy medications like ***cyclophosphamide, paclitaxel, and tamoxifen***. The omega-3 fatty acids in perilla oil may affect drug metabolism, potentially altering treatment outcomes.

- We can minimize the adverse interactions with these drugs by taking no more than 1-2 teaspoons of perilla oil daily, separated from chemotherapy drugs by at least 1 hour. However, it is essential to discuss the use of perilla with our healthcare provider, especially if we are taking medications processed by the liver.

Probiotics:

- Probiotics are beneficial for gut health, but they can interact with immunosuppressive drugs used in cancer treatment, such as *corticosteroids, cyclosporine, and tacrolimus*. Introducing live bacteria while the immune system is compromised could lead to infections.

- To minimize adverse interactions with these drugs, probiotics with high bacterial counts or fermented foods should be avoided within 1-2 hours of taking medication. We should discuss this with our oncologist before using probiotic supplements, particularly if undergoing immunosuppressive therapy.

Turmeric:

The active compound in turmeric, curcumin, is a potent antioxidant and anti-inflammatory agent that may interfere with several chemotherapy drugs, including *cyclophosphamide, doxorubicin, and paclitaxel*, as well as targeted therapy drugs like *imatinib*.

Curcumin's ability to reduce oxidative stress and inflammation can decrease the effectiveness of chemotherapy drugs that rely on these processes to kill cancer cells. Additionally, curcumin may inhibit certain drug transporters and enzymes in drug metabolism, affecting drug availability and efficacy.

To minimize adverse interactions, if you must take the above drugs, take only a tiny amount of turmeric as a spice in food, e.g., ¼ teaspoon per day, at least 2 hours from taking medication. You should also discuss its use with your oncologist to determine appropriate dosages or whether you should avoid it.

Virgin Coconut Oil:

Virgin coconut oil can interact with chemotherapy drugs, such as *cyclophosphamide, doxorubicin, and paclitaxel,* by influencing liver enzymes crucial for drug metabolism, such as the cytochrome P450 enzymes. This interaction may result in altered drug levels in the bloodstream, potentially leading to either reduced effectiveness or increased toxicity. The medium-chain triglycerides (MCTs) in coconut oil can also impact how the body processes and absorbs drugs.

If you must take one of the above drugs, it is safe to take 1-2 teaspoons a day for 1-2 hours after the medication. However, it is important to consult with your oncologist before adding more virgin coconut oil to your regimen during treatment. Of course, you could take your usual dose before and after the treatment.

To make it easier to use the above information, here are **the lists of natural products that may have adverse interactions with each specific drug and products which may have positive interactions and can be used:**

5-Fluorouracil (5-FU) : Avoid *Aloe Arborescens* but can use all the other products from bitter melon to VCO.

Bortezomib (Velcade): Avoid *Blueberries* but can use all the other products from Aloe Arborescens to VCO.

Cisplatin: Avoid *Aloe Arborescens, Bitter Melon, Fucoidan, Garlic, Ginger, Papaya* but we can use Black cumin, Blueberries, Flaxseeds, Mistletoes, Perilla, Probiotics, Turmeric and VCO.

Cyclophosphamide: Avoid *Aloe Arborescens, Flaxseeds, Fucoidan, Garlic, Ginger, Papaya, Perilla, Turmeric, Virgin Coconut Oil.* But we can use Bitter melon, Black cumin, Mistletoes, Probiotics and Honey,

Doxorubicin: Avoid *Aloe Arborescens, Black cumin, Fucoidan, Garlic, Ginger, Papaya, Turmeric, Virgin Coconut Oil.* But we can use Bitter melon, Flaxseeds, Blueberries, Mistletoes, Perilla, Probiotics and Honey.

Erlotinib (Tarceva): Avoid *Blueberries,* But we can use all the other products.

Imatinib: Avoid *Turmeric.* But all the other products can be used with great benefits.

Ipilimumab: Avoid *Honey* . But all the other products can be used with great benefits.

Irinotecan: Avoid *Black cumin.* But all the other products can be used with great benefits.

Letrozole: Avoid *Flaxseeds.* But all the other products can be used with great benefits.

Nivolumab: Avoid *Honey.* But all the other products can be used with great benefits.

Paclitaxel: Avoid *Aloe Arborescens, Bitter melon, Black cumin, Perilla, Turmeric, Virgin Coconut Oil.* But we can use Blueberries, Flaxseeds, Fucoidan, Garlic, Ginger, Mistletoes, Papaya and Probiotics.

Pembrolizumab: Avoid *Honey.* But all the other products can be used with great benefits.

Tamoxifen: Avoid *Blueberries, Flaxseeds and Perilla.* But all the other products can be used.

With Corticosteroids, Cycloporine: and *Tacrolimus: Avoid* Probiotics but we can use all the other products.

NAVIGATING POTENTIAL RISKS - AVOIDING HARMFUL INTER... 109

Common Drugs	Natural Products to avoid the day drugs are taken	Natural Products that can be used anytime
5-Fluorouracil (5-FU)	Aloe Arborescens	All the other products
Bortezomib (Velcade)	Blueberries	All the other products
Cisplatin,	Aloe Arborescens, Bitter melon, Fucoidan, Garlic, Ginger, Papaya	Black cumin, Blueberries, Flaxseeds, Mistletoes, Perilla, Probiotics, Turmeric & VCO
Cyclophosphamide	Aloe Arborescens, Flaxseeds, Fucoidan, Garlic, Ginger, Papaya, Perilla, Turmeric, VCO.	Bitter melon, Black cumin seeds, Mistletoes, Probiotics & Honey
Doxorubicin,	Aloe Arborescens, Black cumin seeds, Fucoidan, Garlic, Ginger, Papaya, Turmeric, VCO.	Bitter melon, Flaxseeds, Blueberries, Mistletoes, Perilla, Honey & Probiotics
Erlotinib (Tarceva0	Blueberries	All the other products
Imatinib	Turmeric	All the other products
Ipilimumab	Honey	All the other products
Irinotecan	Black cumin seeds & Oil	All the other products
Letrozole	Flaxseeds	All the other products
Nivolumab	Honey	All the other products
Paclitaxel	Aloe Arborescens, Bitter Melon, Black cumin seeds, Perilla, Turmeric, VCO.	Blueberries, Flaxseeds, Fucoidan, Garlic, Ginger, Mistletoes, Papaya & Probiotics
Pembrolizumab	Honey	All the other products
Tamoxifen	Blueberries, Flaxseeds and Perilla	All the other products
Cyclosporine, Corticosteroids, And Tacrolimus	Probiotics	All the other products

Table 2: Products to use and not to use with specific cancer drugs

Signs of Negative Reactions

It is essential to know what symptoms to watch for that might indicate an adverse reaction between natural therapies and cancer drugs:

Increased Fatigue or Weakness: This could indicate liver or kidney issues caused by altered drug metabolism.

Unusual Bleeding or Bruising: Certain natural products, like flax seeds and turmeric, have blood-thinning properties that can increase bleeding risk.

Digestive Issues: Nausea, vomiting, or changes in bowel movements may indicate an interaction between a natural product and chemotherapy or targeted therapy.

Skin Changes: Redness, rash, or irritation may occur if a natural product interacts with radiation therapy or certain medications.

If you experience any of these symptoms, seek medical attention and inform your healthcare team about all supplements you take.

Conclusion

While plant-based therapies offer many potential benefits for cancer care, it is essential to navigate these options with caution. Understanding the risks of unwanted interactions between natural therapies with conventional treatments, consulting healthcare professionals, and closely monitoring for any adverse effects can help ensure a safe and effective integrative approach. By taking these steps, we can make informed decisions that support our overall health and improve treatment outcomes. The key is to work collaboratively with healthcare providers to achieve a balanced plan that maximizes benefits while minimizing risks.

References:

1. National Center for Complementary and Integrative Health (NCCIH). (2021). Herbs at a Glance: Potential Interactions with Cancer Treatment. Retrieved from https://nccih.nih.gov

2. American Cancer Society. (2022). Herbs, Botanicals & Other

Products and Their Interactions with Cancer Treatment. Retrieved from https://www.cancer.org

3. Memorial Sloan Kettering Cancer Center (MSKCC). About Herbs, Botanicals & Other Products. Retrieved from https://www.mskcc.org/cancer-care/integrative-medicine/herbs

4. World Health Organization (WHO). (2021). Safety and Interactions of Herbal Medicines in Oncology. Retrieved from https://www.who.int/health-topics/traditional-medicine

5. Tascilar, M., et al. (2006). The Interaction of Herbal Supplements with Chemotherapy in Cancer Patients. Journal of Clinical Oncology, 24(18), 2489-2495.

Chapter 7

Combined Therapies for Common cancers

I am no longer confused and worried but in the future into treatment with clarity and confidence.

Facing a cancer diagnosis can be overwhelming, but finding clarity in your treatment approach can empower you to move forward with confidence. Combining standard medical treatments with plant-based therapies can create a balanced and effective treatment plan tailored specifically for your type of cancer. This chapter provides suggested combined therapies for the following common cancers: Breast cancer, lung cancer, liver cancer, colorectal cancer, pancreatic cancer, prostate cancer, skin cancer (melanoma) and brain cancer. How to prepare and use specific anticancer natural products is also included in this chapter.

Please remember that this is only part of the complete plan of combined therapies, which also require a healthy diet (Chapter 8), and a healthy lifestyle (Chapter 9).

You will notice that what natural anticancer products you can take from one week before surgery to one (low risk- surgery) or two (high risk surgery) weeks after the surgery are same for all types of cancer. They are Honey,

Probiotics and Virgin Coconut oil. All the other products recommended for all types of cancer are not to be taken during that time.

You will also notice that what can be taken during chemotherapy, radiation, targeted therapy and Immunotherapy are almost the same of all types of cancer. Therefore, for cancer other than the common types listed in this chapter, you can have a combined treatment plan similar to the ones listed here, especially as to when and what natural products to take during treatment.

Breast Cancer:

Based on research and clinical studies, the following natural products are selected for breast cancer: Turmeric, Flaxseeds, Black cumin, Bitter melon, Blueberries, Honey, Ginger, Probiotics, Papaya leaves, and virgin coconut oil. We don't have to use all of them at the same time but it is best to use as many as you can for treatment until cancer is cleared.

When combined with conventional treatment some of them may have unwanted interactions as presented in chapter 6. Here is how they can be combined with standard care:

Step one: Once we suspect that we may have breast cancer, or we have been diagnosed with breast cancer and wait for standard treatment, we'd better start taking at least 4 of the above products recommended for breast cancer. Following are their therapeutic dosages;

½ tsp of black cumin seed oil and powder twice a day 10- 30 minutes before meal

1 to 2 cups of fresh or frozen Blueberries a day

1 capsule of turmeric supplement containing 1-2 grams of curcumin a day.

1-2 tablespoons of ground flax seeds with food a day

1 -2 tablespoons of raw or manuka honey a day with food, drink or on its own.

Two 750 mg capsule of Jarrow Formula extract of Bitter melon a day on empty stomach or eat 150 g of boiled bitter melon a day.

1 -2 tablespoons of Virgin Coconut oil daily with food, hot drink or on its own.

1 capsule of 50 Billion CFU probiotics a day such as Innovixlabs Multi-strain Probiotics and 100-200 ml of Greek yogurt or kefir a day

1 -2 slices of fresh ginger (2-3 mm thick) a day with food.

1 -2 cup of dried papaya leaves (1 rounded teaspoon) tea a day between meal for 4-5 week. Take 1 week break and repeat the cycle.

Step 2: Once you know the treatment plan:

Before Surgery:

Some natural products have anticoagulant or hypoglycemic properties. Therefore we have to stop taking the following products a week before surgery: Black cumin, flaxseeds, ginger, papaya leaves tea, ginger, high dose blueberries and bitter melon. However, we can continue taking Honey, Probiotics and Virgin Coconut oil during that time. One or two weeks after he surgery we can resume the previous intake of natural products if there are no other therapies to follow. Consult your doctors before taking them again.

After surgery, when chemotherapy, hormone therapy, targeted therapy or radiation is administered, we have to stop taking natural products that may have unwanted interaction with the treatment drugs from 2 days before to 2 days after the drugs are administered. We can take products that are less likely to have negative interactions. But it is important to let the oncologist know what natural products you take and the timing.

Chemotherapy and radiation:

Most chemotherapy drugs for breast cancer are oxidative stress dependent drugs like doxorubicin, cisplatin. Radiation therapy also rely on oxidative stress effects. Therefore, we have to stop taking natural products that are strong antioxidants during radiation and chemotherapy with oxidative stress dependent drugs such as doxorubicin, paclitaxel, cisplatin.

- Stop taking black cumin, flaxseeds, ginger, papaya leaves tea, bitter melon, virgin coconut oil.

- It is safe to take honey, turmeric, 1/2 cup blueberries a day and probiotics to enhance treatment efficacy and reduce chemotherapy side effects.

If you know the chemotherapy drugs to be used are not oxidative stress dependent such as Erlotinib, Imatinib, Ipilimumab, Irinotecan, Letrozole, Nivolumab, Pembrolizumab, you can look up Table 2 and adjust what you have to stop taking and what you can take. For example, if the drug is Irinotecan, stop taking only Black cumin.

Hormone Therapy

Common Hormone therapy drugs used for breast cancer include Tamoxifen, letrozole, anastrozole, leuprolide, and goserelin. From 2 days before to 2 days after hormone drugs are administered:

- Take only bitter melon, Probiotics and a small amount of honey during hormone therapy.

- Stop taking all the other natural products.

Targeted Therapy

Natural products may interfere with drug metabolism, mechanisms of action or side effects. Some may inhibit or enhance molecular pathways targeted by the therapy unintentionally. Common targeted therapy drugs for breast cancer include Trastuzumab, Palbociclib, Ribociclib and Olaparib.

It is safe to take Honey, Probiotics and Virgin coconut oil during targeted therapy for breast cancer.

Other products can be taken up to 3 days before and 3 days after targeted therapy. However, it is important to let the oncologist know what natural products you take and the timing.

Immunotherapy:

In some cases of breast cancer, immunotherapy is administered with pembrolizumab. During Immunotherapy, we can take, probiotics, virgin coconut oil, papaya leaves tea, and bitter melon and ½ dose of honey.

Step 3: After treatment:

Three days to one week after conventional treatments are complete, we can resume taking all the above until cancer cells or tumors are no longer detected.

****

Lung Cancer

Based on research and clinical studies, the following natural products are selected for Lung cancer: **Aloe arborescens, Bitter melon, Black cumin, Blueberries, Flaxseeds, Garlic, Honey, Probiotics, Papaya leaves, Perilla, Turmeric and Virgin coconut oil. We don't have to use all of them at the same time, but it is best to** but it is best to use as many as you can for treatment until cancer is cleared.

When combined with conventional treatment some of them may have unwanted interactions as presented in chapter 6. Here is how they can be combined with standard care:

Step 1: Once we suspect that we may have lung cancer, or we have been diagnosed with lung cancer and wait for standard treatment, we'd better start taking at least 4 of the above products recommended for lung cancer. Following are their therapeutic dosages:

½ tsp of black cumin seed oil and powder twice a day 10- 30 minutes before meal twice a day

1 to 2 cups of fresh or frozen Blueberries a day

Turmeric supplement containing 1-2 grams of curcumin with meal a day.

1 tablespoon of Aloe Arborescens mixed with raw honey and cognac three times a day 30 minutes before meal. (watch Zago recipe) for 10 days with 10 day-break and repeat the cycle. https://youtu.be/iZtBLFNbhJY?si=cZzA0j815D7B7CBW

1-2 tablespoons of raw honey a day, if Aloe Arborescens is not taken.

1-2 tablespoons of ground flax seeds with food a day

Two 750 mg capsule of Jarrow Formula extract of Bitter melon a day on empty stomach or eat 15o g of boiled bitter melon a day.

1-2 tablespoons of Virgin Coconut oil daily with food, hot drink or on its own.

1 capsule of 50 Billion CFU probiotics a day such as Innovixlabs Multi-strain Probiotics + 100-200 ml of Greek yogurt a day

1-2 slices of fresh ginger (2-3 mm thick) a day with food.

1-2 cups of fresh or frozen blueberries a day,

1-2 cloves of garlic with food a day

1-2 cup of dried papaya leaves (1 rounded tsp) tea a day between meal for 4-5 week. Take 1 week break and repeat the cycle.

Step 2: Once you know the treatment plan:

Before Surgery:

Stop taking the following products 1 weeks before surgery: Aloe Arborescencs, Black cumin, flaxseeds, garlic, papaya leaves tea, Perilla, Bitter melon, Turmeric. However, we can continue taking Honey, Probiotics and Virgin Coconut oil during that time. One or two weeks after he surgery we can resume the previous intake of natural products if there are no other therapies to follow. Consult your doctors before taking them again.

After surgery, when chemotherapy, hormone therapy, targeted therapy or radiation is administered, we have to stop taking natural products that may have unwanted interaction with the treatment drugs from 2 days week before to 2 days after the drugs are administered. We can take products that are less likely to have negative interactions. But it is important to let the oncologist know what natural products you take and the timing.

Chemotherapy and radiation: Most chemotherapy drugs for lung cancer are oxidative stress dependent drugs like doxorubicin, cisplatin, paclitaxel. carboplatin, etoposide. Radiation therapy also rely on oxidative stress effects.

From 2 days before chemotherapy or radiation to 2 days after drugs are administered:

- Stop taking Aloe arborescens, black cumin, flaxseeds, garlic, ginger, bitter melon, turmeric, virgin coconut oil.

- It is safe to take honey, ½ dose of perilla, ½ does of papaya leaves tea, ½ cup of blueberries and 1 capsule of 50 Billon CFU probiotics to enhance treatment efficacy and reduce chemotherapy side effects.

If you know the chemotherapy drugs to be used are not oxidative stress dependent such as Erlotinib, Imatinib, Ipilimumab, Irinotecan, Letrozole, Nivolumab, Pembrolizumab, you can look up Table 2 and adjust what you have to stop taking and what you can take. For example, if the drug is Irinotecan, we only stop taking Black cumin.

Targeted Therapy

Natural products may interfere with drug metabolism, mechanisms of action or side effects. Some may inhibit or enhance molecular pathways targeted by the therapy unintentionally. Common targeted therapy drugs for lung cancer include Erlotinib and Osimertinib, Alectinib, Crizotinib.

It is safe to take Honey, Probiotics and Virgin coconut oil during targeted therapy for lung cancer.

Other products can be taken up to 3 days before and 3 days after targeted therapy. However, it is important to let the oncologist know what natural products you take and the timing.

Immunotherapy: IIn some cases of lung cancer, immunotherapy is administered with Pembrolizumab, or Nivolumab or Atezolizumab. During Immunotherapy, we can *take honey, probiotics, virgin coconut oil, papaya leaves tea, perilla oil/ tea and bitter melon* while stopping all other products..

Step 3: After treatment:

Resume the normal dosage as in Step 1 until cancer is no longer detected.

Liver Cancer

Based on research and clinical studies, the following natural products are selected for liver cancer: Aloe arborescens, Bitter melon, Black cumin, Blueberries, Flaxseeds, Ginger, Honey, Probiotics, Papaya leaves, Turmeric, Perilla oil and leaves. We don't have to use all of them at the same time but it is best to use as many as you can for treatment until cancer is cleared.

When combined with conventional treatment some of them may have unwanted interactions as presented in chapter 6. Here is how they can be combined with standard care:

Step 1: Once we suspect that we may have liver cancer, or we have been diagnosed with liver cancer and wait for standard treatment, we'd better start taking at least 5 of the above products recommended for liver cancer. Following are their therapeutic dosages:

½ tsp of black cumin seed oil and powder twice a day 30 minutes before meal twice a day

1 tablespoon of Aloe Arborescens mixed with raw honey and cognac three times a day 30 minutes before meal. (watch Zago recipe) for 10 days with 10 day-break and repeat the cycle. https://youtu.be/iZtBLFNbhJY?si=cZzA0j815D7B7CBW

1 to 2 cups of fresh or frozen Blueberries a day

1 tablespoon of raw honey a day if Zago recipe mix is not taken.

1-2 tablespoons of ground flax seeds with food a day

Two 750 mg capsule of Jarrow Formula extract of Bitter melon a day on empty stomach or eat 150 g of boiled bitter melon a day.

1 capsule of 50 Billion CFU probiotics a day such as Innovixlabs Multi-strain Probiotics + 100-200 ml of Greek yogurt or kefir a day

1-2 slices of fresh ginger (2-3 mm thick) a day with food.

1-2 cup of dried papaya leaves (1 rounded tsp) tea a day between meal for 4-5 week. Take 1 week break and repeat the cycle.

1 tsp pf perilla oil twice a day with meal.

Turmeric supplement containing 1-2 grams of curcumin with meal a day.

Step 2: Once you know the treatment plan:

Before Surgery: Stop taking the following products 1 weeks before surgery: Aloe Arborescencs, Bitter melon, Black cumin, ginger, Papaya leaves tea, Flaxseeds, Perilla, and Turmeric. However, we can continue taking Honey, Probiotics and Virgin Coconut oil during that time. One or two weeks after he surgery we can resume the previous intake of natural products if there are no other therapies to follow. Consult your doctors before taking them again.

After surgery, when chemotherapy, hormone therapy, targeted therapy or radiation is administered, we have to stop taking natural products that may cause unwanted interactions with treatment drugs or procedure from 2 days before to 2 days after the drugs are administered. We can take products that are less likely to have negative interactions. However, it is important to let the oncologist know what natural products you take and the timing.

Chemotherapy and radiation: Most chemotherapy drugs for liver cancer are oxidative stress dependent drugs like doxorubicin, cisplatin. Radiation therapy also rely on oxidative stress effects. Therefore, we have to stop taking natural products that are strong antioxidants during chemotherapy and radiation therapy. During chemotherapy or radiation therapy:

- Stop taking Aloe arborescens, black cumin, flaxseeds, ginger, bitter melon, turmeric, virgin coconut oil.

- It is safe to take honey , ½ dose of perilla, ½ dose of papaya leaves tea, ½ cup of blueberries a day, and probiotics to enhance treatment efficacy and reduce chemotherapy side effects.

If you know the chemotherapy drugs to be used are not oxidative stress dependent such as Erlotinib, Imatinib, Ipilimumab, Irinotecan, Letrozole, Nivolumab, Pembrolizumab, you can look up Table 2 and adjust what you have to stop taking and what you can take. For example, if the drug is Irinotecan, we only stop taking Black cumin.

Ablation and Embolization: During ablation and embolization procedures for liver cancer, most of anticancer natural products should be avoided because they may interfere with the procedure, wound healing, blood clotting or immune response.

It is safe to take only Honey, Probiotics and Virgin Coconut oil during Ablation and Embolization of the liver.

Targeted Therapy

Natural products may interfere with drug metabolism, mechanisms of action or side effects. Some may inhibit or enhance molecular pathways targeted by the therapy unintentionally. Common targeted therapy drugs for liver cancer include Sorafenib, Lenvatinib, Regorafenib and Cabozantinib.

It is safe to take Honey, Probiotics and Virgin coconut oil during targeted therapy for liver cancer.

Other products can be taken up to 2-3 days before and 2-3 days after targeted therapy. However, it is important to let the oncologist know what natural products you take and the timing.

Immunotherapy: In some cases of liver cancer, immunotherapy is administered with Nivolumab or Atezolizumab with Bevacizumab. During Immunotherapy, we can take honey, probiotics, virgin coconut oil, papaya leaves tea, perilla oil/ tea, ½ cup of blueberries a day and bitter melon while abstaining from the other products.

Step 3: After treatment:

Resume the normal dosage as in Step 1 until cancer is no longer detected.

Colon or Colorectal Cancer

Based on research and clinical studies, the following natural products are selected for Colorectal cancer: **Aloe arborescens, Bitter melon, Black cumin, Blueberries, Garlic, Ginger, Honey, Probiotics, Papaya leaves, Perilla oil and leaves, Turmeric and Virgin coconut oil.** We don't have to use all of them at the same time but it is best to use as many as you can until cancer is cleared.

When combined with conventional treatment some of them may have unwanted interactions as presented in chapter 6. Here is how they can be combined with standard care:

Step 1: Once we suspect that we may have colorectal cancer, or we have been diagnosed with colorectal cancer and wait for standard treatment, we'd better start taking at least 5 of the above products recommended for colorectal cancer. Following are their therapeutic dosages ;

½ tsp of black cumin seed oil and powder twice a day 30 minutes before meal twice a day

Turmeric supplement containing 1-2 grams of curcumin a day.

1 tablespoon of Aloe Arborescens mixed with raw honey and cognac three times a day 30 minutes before meal. (watch Zago recipe) for 10 days with 10 day-break and repeat the cycle. https://youtu.be/iZtBLFNbhJY?si=cZzA0j815D7B7CBW

Two 750 mg capsule of Jarrow Formula extract of Bitter melon a day on empty stomach or eat 15o g of boiled bitter melon a day.

1 tablespoon of raw honey a day if Zago recipe mixture is not taken

1 clove of garlic a day

1 capsule of 50 Billion CFU probiotics a day such as Innovixlabs Multi-strain Probiotics + 100-200 ml of Greek yogurt or kefir a day

1 -2 slices of fresh ginger (2-3 mm thick) a day with food.

1 -2 cup of dried papaya leaves (1 rounded tsp) tea a day between meal for 4-5 week. Take 1 week break and repeat the cycle.

1 tsp of perilla oil and 1 cup of perilla tea twice a day with meal.

2-3 tablespoons of Virgin Coconut Oil a day

1-2 cups of fresh or frozen blueberries a day,

Step 2: Once you know the treatment plan:

Before Surgery: Stop taking the following products 1 weeks before surgery: Aloe Arborescencs, Black cumin, Ginger, Papaya leaves tea, Flaxseeds, Perilla oil, Turmeric. However, we can continue taking Honey, Probiotics and Virgin Coconut oil during that time. One or two weeks after he surgery we can resume the previous intake of natural products if there are no other therapies to follow. Consult your doctors before taking them again.

After surgery, when chemotherapy, hormone therapy, targeted therapy or radiation is administered, we have to stop taking natural products that may cause unwanted interactions with the treatment drugs or procedure from 2 days before to 2 days after the drugs are administered. We can and should take products that are less likely to have negative interactions. But it is important to let the oncologist know what natural products you take and the timing.

Chemotherapy and radiation: Most chemotherapy drugs for colorectal cancer are oxidative stress dependent drugs like 5-FU, capecitabine, oxaliplatin, and irinotecan. Radiation therapy also rely on oxidative stress effects. Therefore, we have to stop taking natural products that are strong antioxidants during chemotherapy and radiation therapy. During chemotherapy:

- Stop taking Aloe arborescens, black cumin, flaxseeds, garlic, ginger, bitter melon, turmeric, virgin coconut oil.

- It is safe to take 1-2 tsp of honey, ½ dose of perilla, ½ does of papaya leaves tea, and probiotics to enhance treatment efficacy and reduce chemotherapy side effects.

If you know the chemotherapy drugs to be used are not oxidative stress dependent such as Erlotinib, Imatinib, Ipilimumab, Irinotecan, Letrozole, Nivolumab, Pembrolizumab, you can look up Table 2 and adjust what you have to stop taking and what you can take. For example, if the drug is Irinotecan, stop taking only Black cumin.

Targeted Therapy

Natural products may interfere with drug metabolism, mechanisms of action or side effects. Some may inhibit or enhance molecular pathways targeted by the therapy unintentionally. Common targeted therapy drugs for colorectal cancer include Cetuximab, Panitumumab, and Bevacizumab.

It is safe to take Honey, Probiotics and Virgin coconut oil during targeted therapy for colorectal cancer.

Other products can be taken up to 2-3 days before and 2-3 days after targeted therapy.

Immunotherapy: In some cases of colorectal cancer, immunotherapy is administered with Nivolumab or Pembrolizumab. During Immunotherapy, we can take honey, probiotics, virgin coconut oil, papaya leaves tea, perilla oil/ tea and bitter melon while abstaining from the other products.

Step 3: After treatment:

Resume the normal dosage as in Step 1 until cancer is no longer detected.

Pancreatic Cancer

Based on research and clinical studies, the following natural products are recommended for pancreatic cancer: Aloe arborescens, Bitter melon, Black cumin, Turmeric, Probiotics, Ginger, Honey, Papaya leaves and Virgin coconut oil. We don't have to use all of them at the same time but it is best to use as many as you can until cancer is cleared.

When combined with conventional treatment some of them may have unwanted interactions as presented in chapter 6. Here is how they can be combined with standard care:

Step 1: Once we suspect that we may have pancreatic cancer, or we have been diagnosed with pancreatic cancer and wait for standard treatment, we'd better start taking at least 4 of the above products recommended for pancreatic cancer. Following are their therapeutic dosages.

• ½ tsp of black cumin seed oil and powder twice a day 30 minutes before meal twice a day

• 1 tablespoon of Aloe Arborescens mixed with raw honey and distillate three times a day 30 minutes before meal. (watch Zago recipe) for 10 days with 10 day-break and repeat the cycle. https://youtu.be/iZtBLFNbhJY?si=cZzA0j815D7B7CBW

• Two 750 mg capsule of Jarrow Formula extract of Bitter melon a day on empty stomach or eat 150 g of boiled bitter melon a day.

• 1 capsule of 50 Billion CFU probiotics a day such as Innovixlabs Multi-strain

• 1 -2 slices of fresh ginger (2-3 mm thick) a day with food.

- 1-2 cup of dried papaya leaves (1 rounded tsp) tea a day between meal for 4-5 week. Take 1 week break and repeat the cycle.

- 1-2 tablespoons Virgin Coconut oil a day with or without foods.

- Turmeric supplement containing 1-2 grams of curcumin.

- 1 tablespoon of raw honey a day, if Zago recipe mix is not taken.

Step 2: Once you know the treatment plan:

Before Surgery: Stop taking the following products 1 weeks before surgery: Aloe Arborescencs, Turmeric, Black cumin, ginger, Papaya leaves tea. However, we can continue taking Honey, Probiotics and Virgin Coconut oil during that time. One or two weeks after he surgery we can resume the previous intake of natural products if there are no other therapies to follow. Consult your doctors before taking them again.

After surgery, when chemotherapy, hormone therapy, targeted therapy or radiation is administered, we have to stop taking natural products that may cause unwanted interactions with the treatment drugs or procedure from 2 days before to 2 days after the drugs are administered. We can and should take products that are less likely to have negative interactions. But it is important to let the oncologist know what natural products you take and the timing.

Chemotherapy and radiation: Most chemotherapy drugs for pancreatic cancer are oxidative stress dependent drugs like Folfirinox – a combination of 5-FU, leucovorin, oxaliplatin, irinotecan -, Gemcitabine, Abraxane, capecitabine, cisplatin, irinotecan, Nab-paclitaxel. Radiation therapy also rely on oxidative stress effects. We have to stop taking natural products that are strong antioxidants during chemotherapy and radiation therapy.

- Stop taking Aloe arborescens, black cumin, flaxseeds, ginger, bitter melon, turmeric, virgin coconut oil.

- It is safe to take 1-2 tsp of honey, ½ dose of perilla, ½ does of papaya leaves tea, and probiotics to enhance treatment efficacy and reduce chemotherapy side effects.

If you know the chemotherapy drugs to be used are not oxidative stress dependent such as Erlotinib, Imatinib, Ipilimumab, Irinotecan, Letrozole, Nivolumab, Pembrolizumab, you can look up Table 2 and adjust what you have to stop taking and what you can take. For example, if the drug is Irinotecan, we only stop taking Black cumin.

Targeted Therapy

Natural products may interfere with drug metabolism, mechanisms of action or side effects. Some may inhibit or enhance molecular pathways targeted by the therapy unintentionally. Common targeted therapy drugs for pancreatic cancer include Erlotinib in combination with gemcitabine, Larotrectinib, Entrectinib.

It is safe to take Honey, Probiotics and Virgin coconut oil during targeted therapy for Pancreatic cancer.

Other products can be taken up to 3 days before and 3 days after targeted therapy.

Immunotherapy: In some cases of pancreatic cancer, immunotherapy is administered with Pembrolizumab. During Immunotherapy, we can take *honey, probiotics, virgin coconut oil, papaya leaves tea, perilla oil/ tea and bitter melon* while abstaining from the other products.

Step 3: After treatment:

Resume the normal dosage as in Step 1 until cancer is no longer detected.

Gastric or Stomach Cancer

Based on research and clinical studies, the following natural products are recommended for gastric or stomach cancer: Black cumin, turmeric, virgin coconut oil, aloe arborescens, honey, ginger, papaya, perilla, probiotics, and bitter melon. We don't have to use all of them at the same time, but it is best to include as many as you can until cancer is cleared.

When combined with conventional treatment some of them may have unwanted interactions as presented in chapter 6. Here is how they can be combined with standard care:

Step 1: Once we suspect that we may have gastric cancer, or we have been diagnosed with gastric cancer and wait for standard treatment, we'd better start taking at least 4 of the above products recommended for gastric cancer. Following are therapeutic doses for the products:

• ½ tsp of black cumin seed oil and powder twice a day 30 minutes before meal twice a day

• 1 tablespoon of Aloe Arborescens mixed with raw honey and distillate three times a day 30 minutes before meal. (watch Zago recipe) for 10 days with 10 day-break and repeat the cycle. https://youtu.be/iZtBLFNbhJY?si=cZzA0j815D7B7CBW

• Two 750 mg capsule of Jarrow Formula extract of Bitter melon a day on empty stomach or eat 150 g of boiled bitter melon a day.

• 1 capsule of 50 Billion CFU probiotics a day such as Innovixlabs Multi-strain

• 1 -2 slices of fresh ginger (2-3 mm thick) a day with food.

- 1-2 cup of dried papaya leaves (1 rounded tsp) tea a day between meal for 4-5 week. Take 1 week break and repeat the cycle.

- 1-2 tablespoons of Virgin coconut oil a day

- 1 cup of perilla tea before meal and 1 tsp of perilla oil twice a day with meal

- Turmeric supplement containing 1 to 2 g of curcumin twice a day.

- 1 tablespoon of raw honey a day if Zago recipe is not taken.

Step 2: Once you know the treatment plan:

Before Surgery: Stop taking the following products 1 weeks before surgery: Aloe Arborescencs, Turmeric, Black cumin, ginger, Papaya leaves tea. However, we can continue taking Honey, Probiotics and Virgin Coconut oil during that time. One or two weeks after he surgery we can resume the previous intake of natural products if there are no other therapies to follow. Consult your doctors before taking them again.

After surgery, when chemotherapy, hormone therapy, targeted therapy or radiation administered, we have to stop taking natural products that may cause unwanted interactions with the treatment drugs or procedure from 2 days before to 2 days after the drugs are administered. We can and should take products that are less likely to have negative interactions. But it is important to let the oncologist know what natural products you take and the timing.

Chemotherapy and radiation: Most chemotherapy drugs for gastric cancer are oxidative stress dependent drugs like 5-FU, capecitabine, cis-platin oxaliplatin, irinotecan. Radiation therapy also rely on oxidative stress effects. We have to stop taking natural products that are strong antioxidants during chemotherapy and radiation therapy. From 2 days before to 2 days after chemotherapy drugs or radiation are administered:

• Stop taking Aloe arborescens, black cumin, flaxseeds, ginger, bitter melon, turmeric, virgin coconut oil.

• Take 1-2 tsp of honey, ½ dose of perilla, ½ does of papaya leaves tea, and probiotics to enhance treatment efficacy and reduce chemotherapy side effects.

If you know the chemotherapy drugs to be used are not oxidative stress dependent such as Erlotinib, Imatinib, Ipilimumab, Irinotecan, Letrozole, Nivolumab, Pembrolizumab, you can look up Table 2 and adjust what you have to stop taking and what you can take. For example, if the drug is Irinotecan, stop taking only Black cumin.

Targeted Therapy

Natural products may interfere with drug metabolism, mechanisms of action or side effects. Some may inhibit or enhance molecular pathways targeted by the therapy unintentionally. Common targeted therapy drugs for gastric cancer are Trastuzumab, Ramucirumab and Pembrozumab.

It is safe to take Honey, Probiotics and Virgin coconut oil during targeted therapy for Gastric cancer.

Other products can be taken up to 2 days before and 2 days after targeted therapy.

Immunotherapy: In some cases of pancreatic cancer, immunotherapy is administered with Pembrolizumab. During Immunotherapy, we can take honey, probiotics, virgin coconut oil, papaya leaves tea, perilla oil/ tea and bitter melon

Other products can be taken up to 2 days before and 2 days after Immunotherapy drug is administered.

Step 3: After treatment:

Resume the normal dosage as in Step 1 until cancer is no longer detected

Prostate Cancer

Based on research and clinical studies, the following natural products are recommended for prostate cancer: **Aloe arborescens, Honey, Blueberries, Papaya leaf and seeds, ginger, Bitter melon, garlic, Turmeric, Black cumin, and flaxseeds.**

We don't have to use all of them at the same time, but it is best to include as many as you can until cancer is cleared.

When combined with conventional treatment some of them may have unwanted interactions as presented in chapter 6. Here is how they can be combined with standard care:

Step 1: Once we suspect that we may have prostate cancer, or we have been diagnosed with prostate cancer and wait for standard treatment, we'd better start taking at least 4 of the above products recommended for prostate cancer. Following are their therapeutic dosages:

• ½ tsp of black cumin seed oil and powder twice a day 30 minutes before meal twice a day

• 1 tablespoon of Aloe Arborescens mixed with raw honey and distillate three times a day 30 minutes before meal. (watch Zago recipe) for 10 days with 10 day-break and repeat the cycle. https://youtu.be/iZtBLFNbhJY?si=cZzA0j815D7B7CBW

• Turmeric supplement containing 1-2 grams of curcumin a day.

• Two 750 mg capsule of Jarrow Formula extract of Bitter melon a day on empty stomach or eat 150 g of boiled bitter melon a day.

• 1 -2 slices of fresh ginger (2-3 mm thick) a day with food.

- 1 clove of garlic with food a day.

- 1-2 cup of dried papaya leaves (1 rounded tsp) tea a day between meal for 4-5 week. Take 1 week break and repeat the cycle.

- 1 tablespoon of honey a day if Zago recipe mix is not taken.

- 1-2 tablespoons of ground flaxseeds with food.

Step 2: Once you know the treatment plan:

Before Surgery: Stop taking the following products 1 weeks before surgery: Aloe Arborescencs, Turmeric, Black cumin, ginger, Papaya leaves tea, bitter melon. However, we can continue taking Honey, Probiotics and Virgin Coconut oil during that time. One or two weeks after he surgery we can resume the previous intake of natural products if there are no other therapies to follow. Consult your doctors before taking them again.

After surgery: when chemotherapy, hormone therapy, targeted therapy or radiation is administered, we have to stop taking natural products that may cause unwanted interactions with the treatment drugs or procedure from 2 days before to 2 days after the drugs are administered. We can and should take products that are less likely to have negative interactions. But it is important to let the oncologist know what natural products you take and the timing.

Chemotherapy and radiation: Most chemotherapy drugs for prostate cancer are oxidative stress dependent drugs like Docetaxel and Cabazitaxel. Radiation therapy also rely on oxidative stress effects. We have to stop taking natural products that are strong antioxidants during chemotherapy and radiation therapy. From 2 days before to 2 days after chemotherapy drugs or radiation are administered:

- Stop taking Aloe arborescens, black cumin, flaxseeds, ginger, bitter melon, turmeric.

- Take probiotics, 1-2 tsp of honey, ½ dose of papaya leaves tea to enhance treatment efficacy and reduce chemotherapy side effects.

If you know the chemotherapy drugs to be used are not oxidative stress dependent such as Erlotinib, Imatinib, Ipilimumab, Irinotecan, Letrozole, Nivolumab, Pembrolizumab, you can look up Table 2 and adjust what you have to stop taking and what you can take. For example, if the drug is Irinotecan, we only stop taking Black cumin.

Targeted Therapy: Natural products may interfere with drug metabolism, mechanisms of action or side effects. Some may inhibit or enhance molecular pathways targeted by the therapy unintentionally. Common targeted therapy drugs for Prostate cancer are Olaparb, Rucaparib.

It is safe to take Honey, Probiotics during targeted therapy for prostate cancer.

Other products can be taken up to 2 days before and 2 days after targeted therapy.

Hormone Therapy: Common hormone drugs used for prostate cancer include leuprolide, goserelin , degarelix and bicalutamide. From 2 days before to 2 days after drugs are administered:

- Take only bitter melon, Probiotics and a small amount of honey.

- Stop taking all the other natural products.

Immunotherapy: In some cases of prostate cancer, immunotherapy is administered with Sipuleucel. During Immunotherapy, we can take honey, probiotics, papaya leaves tea, and bitter melon.

Other products can be taken up to 2 days before and 2 days after Immunotherapy drug is administered.

Step 3: After treatment:

Resume the normal dosage as in Step 1 until cancer is no longer detected.

Brain cancer

Based on research and clinical studies, the following natural products are recommended for Brain cancer: **Aloe arborescens, Honey, Virgin coconut oil, Perilla oil, Ginger, Black cumin, Garlic, Turmeric, Probiotics, Fucoidan.**

We don't have to use all of them at the same time, but it is best to include as many as you can during brain cancer treatment until cancer is cleared.

When combined with conventional treatment some of them may have unwanted interactions as presented in chapter 6. Here are the ways they can be combined with standard care:

Step 1: Once we suspect that we may have brain cancer, or we have been diagnosed with brain cancer and wait for standard treatment, we'd better start taking at least 4 of the above products recommended for prostate cancer. The following are their therapeutic dosages:

• ½ tsp of black cumin seed oil and powder twice a day 30 minutes before meal twice a day

• 1 tablespoon of Aloe Arborescens mixed with raw honey and distillate three times a day 30 minutes before meal. (watch Zago recipe) for 10 days with 10 day-break and repeat the cycle. https://youtu.be/iZtBLFNbhJY?si=cZzA0j815D7B7CBW

• 1-2 tablespoon of honey a day if Zago recipe mixture is not taken.

• Turmeric supplement containing 1-2 grams of curcumin a day.

• 1 -2 slices of fresh ginger (2-3 mm thick) a day with food.

• 1 clove of garlic with food a day.

- 1 cup of perilla tea before meal and 1 tsp of perilla oil with food twice a day

- 2-3 tablespoons of Virgin coconut oil per day with or without food.

- 1 capsule of 50 Billion CFU probiotics a day such as Innovixlabs Multi-strain

- A dose of Fucoidan supplement recommended by manufacturer.

Step 2: Once you know the treatment plan:

Before Surgery: Stop taking the following products 1 weeks before surgery: Aloe Arborescencs, Turmeric, Black cumin, ginger. However, we can continue taking Honey, Probiotics and Virgin Coconut oil during that time. One or two weeks after he surgery we can resume the previous intake of natural products if there are no other therapies to follow. Consult your doctors before taking them again.

After surgery, when chemotherapy, hormone therapy, targeted therapy or radiation is administered, we have to stop taking natural products that may cause unwanted interactions with the treatment drugs or procedure from 2 days before to 2 days after the drugs are administered. We can and should take products that are less likely to have negative interactions. But it is important to let the oncologist know what natural products you take and the timing.

Chemotherapy and radiation: Most chemotherapy drugs for brain cancer are oxidative stress dependent drugs like Temozolomide (an alkylating agent) Radiation therapy also rely on oxidative stress effects. We have to stop taking natural products that are strong antioxidants during chemotherapy and radiation therapy. From 2 days before to 2 days after chemotherapy drugs or radiation are administered:

- Stop taking Aloe arborescens, black cumin, flaxseeds, ginger, turmeric, virgin coconut oil.

- Take probiotics, 1-2 tsp of honey to enhance treatment efficacy and reduce chemotherapy side effects.

If you know the chemotherapy drugs to be used are not oxidative stress dependent such as Erlotinib, Imatinib, Ipilimumab, Irinotecan, Letrozole, Nivolumab, Pembrolizumab, you can look up Table 2 and adjust what you have to stop taking and what you can take. For example, if the drug is Irinotecan, we only stop taking Black cumin.

Targeted Therapy: Natural products may interfere with drug metabolism, mechanisms of action or side effects. Some may inhibit or enhance molecular pathways targeted by the therapy unintentionally. Common targeted therapy drug for brain cancer is Bevacizumab.

It is safe to take Honey, Probiotics during targeted therapy for Brain cancer.. Other products can be taken up to 2 days before and 2 days after targeted therapy.

Immunotherapy: In some cases of brain cancer, immunotherapy is administered with pembrolizumab. During Immunotherapy:

We can take honey, probiotics, papaya leaves tea, and bitter melon

Other products can be taken up to 2 days before and 2 days after Immunotherapy drug is administered.

Step 3: After treatment:

Resume the normal dosage as in Step 1 until cancer is no longer detected.

Skin Cancer (Melanoma)

Based on research and clinical studies, the following natural products are recommended for Skin cancer: **Turmeric, Virgin coconut oil, Aloe arborescens, Blueberries, Manuka Honey, Black cumin, Bitter melon, Perilla, Probiotics, and Fucoidan**. We don't have to use all of them at the same time, but it is best to use as many of them as possible until cancer is cleared.

When combined with conventional treatment some of them may have unwanted interactions as presented in chapter 6. Here is how they can be combined with standard care:

Step 1: Once we suspect that we may have skin cancer, or we have been diagnosed with skin cancer and wait for standard treatment, we'd better start taking at least 5 of the above products recommended for liver cancer. The following are their therapeutic dosages;

- ½ tsp of black cumin seed oil and powder twice a day 30 minutes before meal twice a day

- 1 tablespoon of Aloe Arborescens mixed with raw honey and cognac three times a day 30 minutes before meal. (watch Zago recipe) for 10 days with 10 day-break and repeat the cycle. https://youtu.be/iZtBLFNbhJY?si=cZzA0j815D7B7CBW

- 1 tablespoon of raw manuka honey a day if Zago recipe mix is not taken.

- Two 750 mg capsule of Jarrow Formula extract of Bitter melon a day on empty stomach or eat 150 grams of boiled bitter melon a day.

- 1 capsule of 50 Billion CFU probiotics a day such as Innovixlabs Multi-strain Probiotics + 100-200 ml of Greek yogurt or kefir a day

- 1 cup of perilla leaves tea before meal and 1 tsp pf perilla oil twice a day with meal.

- Turmeric supplement containing 1-2 grams of curcumin with meal a day.

- 2-3 tablespoons of virgin coconut oil a day with or without food.

- 1 dose of Fucoidan per day as suggested by the producer.

- 1-2 cup of fresh or frozen blueberries a day.

Step 2: Once you know the treatment plan:

Before Surgery: Stop taking the following products 1 week before surgery: Aloe Arborescens, Bitter melon, Black cumin, Perilla, Ginger, Fucoidan, and Turmeric. However, we can continue taking Honey, Probiotics and Virgin Coconut oil during that time. One or two weeks after he surgery we can resume the previous intake of natural products if there are no other therapies to follow. Consult your doctors before taking them again.

After surgery, when chemotherapy, hormone therapy, targeted therapy or radiation is administered, we have to stop taking natural products that may cause unwanted interactions with treatment drugs or procedure from 2 days before to 2 days after the drugs are administered. We can take products that are less likely to have negative interactions. However, it is important to let the oncologist know what natural products you take and the timing.

Chemotherapy and radiation: Most chemotherapy drugs for skin cancer are oxidative stress dependent drugs like Cisplatin combined with Vinblastine, Dacarbazine, Temozolomide. Radiation therapy also rely on oxidative stress effects. Therefore, we have to stop taking natural products that are strong antioxidants during chemotherapy and radiation therapy. During chemotherapy or radiation therapy:

• Stop taking Aloe arborescens, black cumin, ginger, bitter melon, turmeric, Fucoidan and virgin coconut oil.

• It is safe to take honey, perilla and probiotics to enhance treatment efficacy and reduce chemotherapy side effects.

If you know the chemotherapy drugs to be used are not oxidative stress dependent such as Erlotinib, Imatinib, Ipilimumab, Irinotecan, Letrozole, Nivolumab, Pembrolizumab, you can look up Table 2 and adjust what you have to stop taking and what you can take. For example, if the drug is Irinotecan, stop taking only Black cumin.

Targeted Therapy

Natural products may interfere with drug metabolism, mechanisms of action or side effects. Some may inhibit or enhance molecular pathways targeted by the therapy unintentionally. Common targeted therapy drugs for skin cancer include Vemurafenib, Dabrafenib, Trametinib and Cobimetinib.

It is safe to take Honey, Probiotics and Virgin coconut oil during targeted therapy for skin cancer.

Other products can be taken up to 2 days before and 2 days after targeted therapy. However, it is important to let the oncologist know what natural products you take and the timing.

Immunotherapy:

In some cases of skin cancer, immunotherapy is administered with Pembrolizumab, Nivolumab and Ipilimumab. From 2 days before to 2 days after these drugs are administered, we can take honey, probiotics, virgin coconut oil, papaya leaves tea, perilla oil/ tea and bitter melon while abstaining from the other products.

Step 3: After treatment:

Resume the normal dosage as in Step 1 until cancer is no longer detected.

How these natural products are prepared and used.

We will now explore how to use the natural products, their dosage, and the duration of use as recommended by clinicians and research, according to the information provided by cancer support and research organizations.

Aloe arborescens: 10 – 30 ml of aloe juice extract daily, when none of the following drugs: *Doxorubicin, Cisplatin, Cyclophosphamide, and 5-Fluorouracil (5-FU)* is taken.

The best way is to combine aloe arborescens with honey and some distillate. This Brazilian folk recipe is publicized in Father Zago's book "Cancer can be cured." This mixture consists of 2-3 aloe arborescens leaves from over 5-year-old plants, picked before sunrise or after sunset, to be immediately blended with half a kilo of raw honey and three or four tablespoons of distillate (eg. Rum, Cognac with 40% alcohol). Before mixing, we should clean the leaves with a dry cloth, remove their spines, and cut them into pieces. It is recommended that to cure cancer, we take one tablespoons three times a day before meals for 10 days, then stop for 10 days, retake it for another 10 days, and repeat the cycle until wholly cured. For prevention, we should take one tablespoon three times a day, for ten days, at least once a year.

Bitter melon: 50-500 mL of bitter melon juice or 500mg of extract daily when none of *cisplatin, doxorubicin or similar drugs* is taken.

We can consume Bitter melon in several forms, including fresh juice, tea, capsules, or cooked as part of a meal. Its bitter taste may be off-putting to some, but we can combine it with other fruits or vegetables in smoothies to improve its palatability. To further reduce its bitterness, we can soak bitter melon in salt water before cooking or prepare it with sweet ingredients to balance the flavor. Some people also use bitter melon extract as a supplement, which provides a concentrated dose of its active compounds. Bitter melon tea is another popular way to consume this fruit, using dried slices of the fruit or ready-made tea bags.

Bitter melon juice: Start with 50ml (2-3 tablespoons) of fresh juice daily diluted with water, early in the morning on an empty stomach. Gradually increase to 200ml if tolerated well.

Bitter melon tea: Brew 1-2 teaspoons of dried bitter melon pieces or 1 tea bag brewed in hot water for 5-10 minutes. Drink 1-2 cup daily after meals.

Bitter melon extract: 500-1000mg per day in divided dose with meals.

Black cumin: When none of *cyclophosphamide, doxorubicin, and paclitaxel i*s taken, we can take 4 to 10 grams of black cumin seed oil daily for 4 to 8 weeks. It is best to start with 2 ml or half a teaspoon twice a day with meals. This dosage is also safe for extended periods. At the same time, take 1-2 grams of seeds (or ½ tsp) twice daily with food as the seeds have more bioactive compounds that heal your whole body. The seeds can also be ground and used as a cooking spice, adding flavor and medicinal value to your meals. They have a distinct, slightly peppery taste that can enhance a variety of dishes, from soups and stews to roasted vegetables and breads. We can take ground black cumin seeds with honey or yogurt, which provides an easy way to incorporate their health benefits into your diet. As it has blood thinning property, we should stop taking it at least 2 weeks before any surgical operation.

Blueberries: A typical recommendation is around 1 to 2 cups of fresh or frozen blueberries per day (about 75-150 grams) when none of *Tamoxifen, Irinotecan, Erlotinib (Tarceva), Cyclophosphamide, Bortezomib (Velcade) i*s taken.

Flaxseeds: When *tamoxifen or letrozole i*s not taken, you can eat 1-2 tablespoons of ground flaxseeds daily. You can mix them with porridge, yogurt, and soup or sprinkle them on roast vegetables.

Fucoidan is usually available in capsule form. Take 500mg to 1 gram daily for 4-8 weeks when none of *cisplatin or doxorubicin or cyclophosphamide* is taken.

Garlic: Take 1-2 cloves of garlic with food or one capsule of aged garlic extract daily when none of *cyclophosphamide, or doxorubicin, or cisplatin or blood thinners* is taken.

Ginger: 3-5 grams of fresh or 1-2 grams dried ginger daily with food when none of *cyclophosphamide, doxorubicin and blood thinners is taken.*

Honey: 1 tablespoon of raw or manuka honey daily when none of *pembrolizumab, nivolumab, and ipilimumab.* is taken. Another way to incorporate honey into your routine is by mixing it with turmeric or ginger, which have additional anti-inflammatory and antioxidant effects, creating a powerful natural remedy to support overall health. But the best is to be part of the aloe arborescens honey mixture described above with Aloe Arborescens..

Mistletoe extract: often administered 2-3 times per week via subcutaneous injection and under medical supervision. It needs to be added to the recommended list due to its complexity. If you want to use mistletoe extract, it is best to consult a healthcare provider who is familiar with it.

Papaya: We can use papaya leaf juice, papaya leaf tea or papaya seeds when *cyclophosphamide or doxorubicin is not taken.*

Papaya Leaf Juice: Take 20-50 mL of fresh papaya leaf juice per day on an empty stomach in the morning . Start with a smaller dose (around 10-15 mL) and gradually increase to avoid potential side effects like nausea.

Papaya Leaf Tea: Dosage: Boil 1 teaspoon of dried crumbled Papaya leaves in 250 -300 mL of water. Drink 1-2 cups when still warm between meals for best absorption. Take a week break after 4-5 weeks.

Papaya Leaf Extract/Capsules: Take around 500 mg to 1,000 mg per day with water, ideally before meals. Papaya leaf can be used long-term, but if we use it alongside conventional treatment, we should discuss the optimal duration with our oncologist to avoid interactions.

Papaya Seeds: Papaya seeds can be eaten raw directly or as ground powder, or consumed dried as a powder added to food or taken with water:

With raw seeds, we can start with 1-2 teaspoons (or 10-15 seeds) of raw papaya seeds per day. They have a strong, peppery taste, so we can take them with honey or add them to smoothies. We can chew the seeds or grind them into a powder to mix with food or drinks once or twice daily.

Dried Papaya Seeds: To save the seeds when eating papaya fruits, we can dry them in the sun or a dehydrator and grind them before using them. We can start with one teaspoon of the powder daily on salads, soups, smoothies, and yogurt and increase it to two teaspoons daily with close monitoring of its effects.

We should take Papaya seeds in cycles, such as 2-3 weeks of use followed by a break of 1-2 weeks. This cycling helps avoid digestive upset or any long-term side effects. As part of a supportive regimen, use for 3-6 months, then reassess with a healthcare professional to decide whether to continue.

Caution: Papaya seeds and leaves are generally not recommended for pregnant women due to their potential effects on the uterus

Perilla: One teaspoon of perilla oil twice daily or a cup of perilla leaves (1 tsp) tea twice a day is recommended when *cyclophosphamide, paclitaxel, and tamoxifen* are not used .

Perilla oil can be drizzled over salads or added to smoothies, providing an easy way to incorporate this nutrient-dense oil into your diet. Perilla leaves can also be consumed as part of a salad, used in cooking, or brewed into tea. They can also be added to soups and stir-fries, offering a unique flavor and therapeutic benefits. Perilla leaves have a distinctive aroma and taste that make them a popular ingredient in Asian cuisine, and their nutritional benefits make them an excellent addition to a cancer-supportive diet.

Probiotics: Daily intake of probiotics supplements or fermented foods such as live yogurt, kefir, Kimchi, Sauerkraut when *corticosteroids, cyclosporine, and tacrolimus are* not taken.

Turmeric: When *cyclophosphamide, doxorubicin, paclitaxel, imatinib and similar drugs* are not taken, we can take a turmeric supplement with piperine (for enhanced absorption) containing 500 mg to 2 grams of curcumin daily or 10 to 30 grams of lakadong turmeric powder with 1-2 grams of black pepper (for enhanced absorption) a day.

We can incorporate turmeric powder into our diet by using it as a spice in cooking, such as in curries, soups, and stews, or turmeric tea with a pinch of black pepper to enhance its absorption. We can add turmeric to smoothies, golden milk (a warm beverage made with milk and turmeric), or sprinkle it on roasted vegetables. Another great way to incorporate turmeric is by making turmeric paste, also known as "golden paste," which can be added to various dishes or taken directly for a concentrated health boost.

Turmeric can also be combined with other beneficial spices to create an anti-inflammatory blend that can be used in a variety of recipes. For example, combining turmeric with ginger can provide synergistic benefits that may help reduce cancer-related inflammation and discomfort. Adding cinnamon not only enhances the flavor but also provides additional antioxidants, further supporting the body's defense mechanisms.

Virgin coconut oil: Take 1-2 tablespoons daily when *cyclophosphamide, doxorubicin, paclitaxel and similar drugs* are not taken.. You can take it directly or with coffee, tea, soup, porridge, warm water or spread on toast.

Chapter 8

Nutrition and Diet: Fueling Your Fight

Nutrition plays a crucial role in supporting cancer treatment and recovery. A well-balanced diet can strengthen your body during cancer treatment, provide much-needed energy, and reduce side effects like nausea, fatigue, and weakness. Consuming nutrient-rich foods can also help boost your immune system, making it easier for your body to fight infections and recover more effectively. Proper nutrition can improve both physical and mental health, which is vital during such a challenging time. A healthy diet is one of the common secrets of cancer survivors. This chapter will explore the importance of diet and nutrition for cancer patients, focusing on foods that support treatment and those best avoided, along with practical meal plans to help maintain a balanced diet.

Foods to Avoid

Research from organizations like the World Cancer Research Fund and other cancer organizations certain foods can hinder the effectiveness of cancer treatments or increase side effects and should be avoided.

Processed Foods: Foods high in preservatives, additives, and unhealthy fats can negatively impact the immune system and overall health. Limit the consumption of processed snacks, ready-made meals, and fast food. Processed meats, canned foods with high sodium content, and packaged snacks often contain unhealthy additives that can impair immune function. Red meat and processed foods have been linked to an increased risk of cancer progression.

When we are severely sick, especially during cancer treatment, our friends and relatives may give us Ensure, a nutritional supplement drink. However, it may not be suitable for cancer patients. Its high sugar content could impact inflammation and insulin. It contains artificial flavors and preservatives, which make it unhealthy. Its ingredients, like dairy or soy, might cause gas or bloating, especially during chemotherapy. It may also lack sufficient protein and nutrients for muscle maintenance and healing.

Sugar: High sugar intake can lead to insulin spikes and inflammation, which may contribute to cancer progression. Reduce the consumption of sugary beverages, candies, and desserts. Sugary foods and drinks, including Ensure, should be minimized, as high sugar intake can contribute to inflammation and interfere with the body's ability to recover

Alcohol: Alcohol can weaken the immune system, interact with medications, and potentially worsen the side effects of cancer treatment. It is best to avoid alcohol during treatment.

By avoiding the above foods, we actually starve cancer cells of their preferred energy source.

Foods to Support Cancer Treatment

Research from organizations like the World Cancer Research Fund and other cancer organizations has shown that certain foods can aid in cancer treatment. As a result, The World Health Organization (WHO) recommends consumption of following foods during cancer treatment and for cancer prevention:

1. **Colorful Fruits and Vegetables.** These foods contain essential vitamins, minerals, and antioxidants that help combat oxidative stress, a condition often exacerbated by cancer treatments. Antioxidants can also help reduce inflammation, thereby supporting the healing process. Foods like berries, leafy greens, carrots, broccoli, sweet potatoes and citrus fruits are rich in antioxidants such as vitamin C, vitamin E, and beta-carotene, which are vital for immune function.

2. **Lean Proteins**: Lean proteins, including poultry, fish, beans, hemp seeds, mushrooms, and low-fat dairy products, are recommended to help repair tissues and maintain muscle mass during treatment. Protein is especially important for patients undergoing chemotherapy or radiation, as these treatments can lead to muscle loss and increased fatigue. Protein-rich foods also support immune function, which is critical for patients whose immune systems may be compromised by treatment.

3. **Whole Grains**: Whole grains like brown rice, quinoa, oats, and whole-wheat bread are rich in fiber, vitamins, and minerals. They help regulate blood sugar levels, maintain energy, and support gut health. Fiber also plays a crucial role in preventing constipation, which is a common side effect of certain cancer treatments.

4. **Healthy Fats**: Incorporating healthy fats such as omega-3 fatty acids, which are found in fatty fish (e.g., salmon and mackerel),

flaxseeds, chia seeds, hemp seeds and walnuts with anti-inflammatory properties can help minimize inflammation caused by cancer treatments and reduce treatment-related fatigue.

5. **Hydration**: Adequate hydration is essential. Drinking plenty of water helps flush toxins out of the body and prevent dehydration, which can be a common side effect of chemotherapy and radiation.

6. **Anti-Inflammatory Foods:** Turmeric, ginger, garlic, yogurt and green tea have anti-inflammatory properties that can support the body during treatment and reduce side effects. Turmeric contains curcumin, a powerful anti-inflammatory compound. Ginger, garlic, and green tea also reduce inflammation and support the immune system during treatment.

Meal time and meal size

Research has shown that intermittent fasting for 14-16 hours a day may play a supportive role in cancer treatment by improving metabolic health and reducing inflammation. Fasting is one of the common habits of cancer survivors. It is therefore beneficial to separate the last meal of the previous day and the first meal of the day by 14 to 16 hours. For example, if you finish your dinner at 6 pm and no snacks in the evening, then you should have breakfast only after 8 am. It helps lower insulin levels and blood sugar, potentially starving cancer cells of their preferred energy source. Such fasting may also enhance the body's response to treatments by promoting cellular repair processes and boosting immune function.

Avoiding eating until full is important because overloading the digestive system can cause oxidative stress and inflammation, which may hinder the body's ability to fight cancer. Instead, moderate (less than 80% full), nutrient-dense meals can provide essential nutrients without burdening the body.

Benefits of the of healthy diet for cancer treatment

The above well-balanced diet as recommended by the WHO can help enhance the effectiveness of cancer treatments, minimize adverse effects, and improve quality of life in several ways:

Enhancing the effectiveness of cancer treatment:

- **Supporting Immune Function**: A diet rich in antioxidants and nutrients helps boost the immune system, making the body more capable of fighting cancer cells and infections that may arise during treatment.

- **Improving Energy Levels**: Whole grains, lean proteins, and healthy fats help maintain consistent energy levels, allowing patients to better withstand the physical toll of treatments like chemotherapy and radiotherapy.

- **Reducing Inflammation**: Omega-3 fatty acids and antioxidants found in fruits, vegetables, and healthy fats help reduce inflammation, which can improve the effectiveness of treatments by creating an environment that is less conducive to tumor growth.

Minimizing adverse effects

- **Managing Gastrointestinal Symptoms**: Fiber from whole grains, fruits, and vegetables helps prevent constipation and supports a healthy gut. Probiotic-rich foods like yogurt can also help balance gut bacteria, reducing gastrointestinal side effects such as diarrhea.

- **Reducing Nausea and Vomiting**: Ginger, bananas, and small, frequent meals can help mitigate nausea and vomiting caused by chemotherapy.

- **Preventing Malnutrition**: Cancer patients often experience a loss of appetite. Including nutrient-dense, calorie-rich foods like avocados, nuts, and smoothies can help patients meet their nutritional needs and avoid weight loss.

Improving Quality of Life

A healthy diet also plays a vital role in improving the overall quality of life for cancer patients:

- **Maintaining Muscle Mass**: Lean proteins and strength-boosting foods help patients maintain muscle mass, reducing fatigue and improving mobility.

- **Enhancing Mental Health**: Proper nutrition supports brain health, helping to alleviate anxiety and depression. Omega-3 fatty acids are particularly known for their positive impact on mood regulation and cognitive function.

- **Boosting Recovery**: By providing essential vitamins and minerals, the WHO-recommended diet supports faster recovery and better tolerance to ongoing treatments.

Testimonials from Cancer Patients

Many cancer patients have reported significant improvements in their well-being after following WHO's dietary recommendations.

- Maria, a breast cancer survivor, said, "Switching to a diet full of fruits, vegetables, and lean proteins made a noticeable difference. I felt more energized, and my body seemed to handle chemotherapy much better."

- John, who underwent treatment for colon cancer, shared, "The focus on whole grains and healthy fats really helped my digestion and reduced the fatigue I was experiencing. I could feel my body getting stronger."

- Sarah, a patient in remission, stated, "Proper hydration and avoiding processed foods helped me feel less bloated and more comfortable during radiation treatment. My quality of life improved a lot thanks to these small dietary changes."

Practical Meal Plans and Tips for Maintaining a Balanced Diet

- **Focus on Variety:** Aim to consume a colorful variety of fruits and vegetables, lean proteins, whole grains, and healthy fats to ensure you receive a wide range of nutrients.

- **Small, Frequent Meals**: Eating smaller meals more frequently can help manage side effects like nausea and ensure you get enough calories to maintain energy.

- **Stay Hydrated**: Proper hydration is critical to managing treatment side effects like dry mouth, fatigue, and constipation. Drink plenty of water, herbal teas, and clear broths throughout the day.

Meal Planning:

Sample Daily and Weekly Meal Plans for Cancer Patients.

Daily Meal Plan

Example

- **Breakfast**: Oatmeal topped with blueberries, chia seeds, black cumin seeds, and a drizzle of honey. Green tea on the side.

- **Morning Snack**: Greek yogurt with sliced strawberries and a handful of walnuts.

- **Lunch**: Grilled salmon (or tofu and mushroom) with quinoa and steamed broccoli seasoned with turmeric and black pepper.

- **Afternoon Snack**: Sliced cucumber and bell peppers with hummus.

- **Dinner**: Baked chicken breast (or tofu) with roasted sweet potatoes, sautéed spinach, garlic, and black cumin seeds.

- **Evening Snack**: Herbal tea with a small handful of almonds.

Weekly Meal Plan Example

- **Monday**: Serve quinoa salad with mixed greens, cherry tomatoes, avocado, and grilled tofu, along with a side of ginger-carrot soup.

- **Tuesday**: Baked cod with brown rice and roasted Brussels sprouts. Snack on an apple with almond butter.

- **Wednesday**: Lentil stew with turmeric, cumin, carrots, and kale. Serve with whole-grain bread.

- **Thursday**: Stir-fried vegetables (bell peppers, snap peas, mushrooms) with tofu over soba noodles. Sprinkle with sesame seeds.

- **Friday**: Grilled shrimp with wild rice and steamed asparagus. For dessert, a smoothie with spinach, banana, and flax seeds.

- **Saturday**: Turkey and vegetable chili with black beans, tomatoes, and bell peppers. Serve with a small side of guacamole (avocado-based dip) and whole-grain chips.

- **Sunday**: A veggie-packed omelet with spinach, mushrooms, and tomatoes. Serve with a slice of whole-grain toast and fresh orange slices.

Conclusion

Proper nutrition can be vital in supporting cancer treatment and improving recovery. By focusing on nutrient-dense foods, reducing processed foods, sugar, and alcohol, and following a well-balanced meal plan, you can support your body and improve your overall well-being during treatment. Always work with your healthcare provider or a nutrition specialist to create a diet plan that is right for you, ensuring that your nutrition choices effectively support your treatment journey.

References:

1. World Health Organization. (2022). Healthy Diet Fact Sheet. Retrieved from https://www.who.int/news-room/fact-sheets/detail/healthy-diet

2. American Cancer Society. (2021). Nutrition for People with Cancer. Retrieved from https://www.cancer.org/cancer/survivo

rship-during-and-after-treatment/nutrition

3. National Cancer Institute. (2020). Eating Hints: Before, During, and After Cancer Treatment. Retrieved from https://www.cancer.gov/publications/patient-education/eating-hints

Chapter 9

Mind and Body Healing: Finding Strength from Within

Believe, hope, and move forward confidently—your mindset can be your greatest ally in the fight against cancer.

Facing cancer can be an emotionally challenging journey, filled with fear, anxiety, and Stress. However, cultivating a positive mindset rooted in belief, hope, and confidence can significantly impact your experience and outcome during treatment. This chapter explores the power of a positive attitude, stress-reduction techniques, and practical ways to nurture your emotional well-being during treatment, supported by testimonials and clinical evidence.

Believing, Hoping, and Staying Confident

Many people have defeated cancer, even from the advanced stages of the deadliest types. Despite being told they had little time left, they chose not to accept the prognosis. Instead, they fought for their lives, never giving up. Their main secret was unwavering belief in the body's healing power in suitable environment and confidence in their ability to overcome cancer. This belief, combined with faith and hope, helped them fight against the disease, replacing fear, anxiety, stress, and despair with strength and determination.

A strong mindset can profoundly influence your journey through cancer treatment. Studies have shown that patients who maintain a hopeful and positive attitude are often better able to manage side effects, stick to their treatment plans, and even experience improved outcomes. Testimonials from cancer survivors emphasize the importance of hope in their journeys:

Sarah's Story:

Sarah was diagnosed with breast cancer when she was 45. She credits her successful recovery to her determination to stay positive, attend support groups, and practice daily affirmations. Sarah shares that believing in herself and focusing on hope allowed her to face each treatment session with courage.

Clinical Evidence: Studies suggest that positive emotions can lower levels of stress hormones like cortisol, leading to better immune function. Patients who actively cultivate hope and confidence show fewer symptoms of anxiety and depression, which contributes to better overall well-being during treatment.

The Importance of Reducing Stress

Stress has a significant impact on both physical and mental health. High levels of Stress can impair immune function, increase inflammation, and interfere with the body's ability to heal. Therefore, managing stress effectively is crucial during cancer treatment:

Reduced Cortisol Levels: Studies have shown that stress-reduction techniques such as meditation and breathing exercises can lower cortisol levels. Lower cortisol levels are associated with improved immune function, which is critical for cancer patients.

Improved Quality of Life: Patients who engage in relaxation techniques and physical activity report an enhanced quality of life, reduced fatigue, and an improved ability to cope with treatment challenges. Stress reduction helps patients stay on track with treatment schedules and improves adherence to medical recommendations.

Cultivating Hope, Confidence, and Calm

Faith plays a vital role in healing by providing emotional resilience, hope, and community support. Many find that faith reduces stress, helping them stay calm and positive, which can aid physical recovery. For instance, Mary, a cancer survivor, noted that prayer eased her fears, while Carlos, who overcame leukemia, said his faith gave him the strength to persevere. Faith-based communities also offer crucial support, reducing feelings of loneliness. Additionally, faith helps many accept their illness, promoting coping and peace, as seen with John, who lives with Parkinson's. Studies like those in the Journal of Religion and Health show that patients with strong spiritual beliefs often experience better emotional well-being and a greater sense of purpose. Belief in something greater can bring comfort even when physical healing isn't possible, easing fears about death and improving quality of life. For more insights, resources like Harold Koenig's The Healing Power of Faith and articles in the Journal of Religion and Health offer deeper understanding.

I have an experience of faith I would like to share with you.

In April 2021, I was diagnosed with sepsis, a severe blood infection. After one week in the hospital, the hospital cardiologists told me and my family they could not do anything to save me because it is impossible to get rid of bacteria colonizing my pig tissue mitral valve except by replacing it, which is too risky for my damaged lungs, kidneys liver and hearts. Only by a miracle could I survive. All they could do was to help me die without pain. A week later, they sent me home with a supply of IV antibiotics for six weeks, but they did not have any hope for me.

I did not take the prognosis seriously. I was not frightened or worried. I felt calm, knowing that God would take care of me. I felt the presence of God and knew that everything would be OK. Thanks to God's guidance, I learned that Propolis, Zinc, and Selenium supplements would help me in the battle against sepsis. I started taking them in the hospital and continued for many months to strengthen my immune system to fight the infection alongside antibiotics. After finishing the antibiotics, I went to see the hospital infection specialist. He told me the infection had cleared, and my liver, lungs, and kidneys had returned to normal. And here I am now (November 2024) in good health.

Emotional Resilience

Emotional resilience is adapting to challenges and maintaining hope during adversity. Here are some techniques to build resilience:

Affirmations: Affirmations are positive, intentional statements that help shape beliefs and influence the subconscious mind. Repeating affirmations can create a sense of inner calm and focus, which is particularly helpful in stressful situations like cancer treatment. Here's how they work:

- **Shift in Focus**: Affirmations encourage the mind to focus on strengths, hope, and positivity, which can be uplifting during moments of uncertainty or fear.

- **Neural Conditioning**: Repeating affirmations reinforces positive thought patterns, creating new neural pathways that make it easier to think optimistically over time.

- **Stress Reduction**: Positive affirmations can reduce cortisol levels, minimize Stress, and boost resilience. This effect benefits patients as reducing Stress can improve mood, boost immune response, and increase overall mental well-being.

- **Confidence Building**: By focusing on empowering statements, affirmations can cultivate a belief in one's ability to cope, fostering confidence in treatment and healing.

Repeating positive affirmations such as " God has a plan and purpose for me," " This illness is a wake-up call for a change in my diet and lifestyle," "I am strong," and "I can help my body heal with a better diet and lifestyle" "I am healing," or "I have the power to get through this," "I trust in my body's ability to heal and recover every day," "I accept my body as it is and trust in the process of healing," and "I embrace each day's journey, knowing it leads me closer to health" can help instill confidence and reduce fear.

Support Networks: Engage with support groups, family, and friends. Sharing your journey and hearing the stories of others can provide hope and strength, reminding you that you are not alone.

Mindfulness: Mindfulness involves focusing on the present moment and accepting it without judgment. It helps reduce anxiety about the future and fosters a calm and hopeful state of mind. Meditation, deep breathing, visualization of body parts, and energy flow can help you achieve mindfulness.

MIND AND BODY HEALING: FINDING STRENGTH FROM WITHIN 169

Gratitude has a profound impact on mental well-being, boosting immune function and often enhancing resilience, happiness, and even physical health.

Reducing Stress and anxiety: Practicing gratitude encourages the brain to focus on positive experiences, which can diminish Stress and anxiety. Acknowledging what we are grateful for shifts attention from negative emotions to positive thoughts, creating a sense of peace.

Improving mood: Gratitude activates the brain's reward centers, releasing neurotransmitters like dopamine and serotonin, which are associated with happiness and satisfaction. This neural shift can boost mood and counteract symptoms of depression.

Enhancing resilience: Recognizing things to be grateful for, especially during tough times, helps build resilience. This mindset can make it easier to handle adversity, as people often find strength in recognizing the support, resources, or opportunities still available to them.

Strengthening relationship: Expressing gratitude toward others fosters connection and improves relationships, creating a social support network that enhances well-being. People who regularly express appreciation tend to have more positive interactions, which boosts their overall mental and emotional health.

Improving self-esteem and confidence: Gratitude helps reduce the tendency to compare oneself to others, focusing instead on personal blessings and achievements. This focus can increase self-esteem and satisfaction, leading to a healthier self-image and confidence.

Here are some stories and studies illustrating the impact of gratitude:

- On National Public Radio (NPR), Katie, who is in remission from cancer, described how keeping a gratitude list gave her a new perspective on life. Even during painful treatments, she found things to appreciate, which helped her stay motivated and uplifted.

- Michael, a heart disease survivor, shared with *American Heart Association News* that gratitude practices improved his heart health and reduced stress.

- Laura, a chronic illness survivor, shared in *Psychology Today* that gratitude journaling helped her cope with tough days, providing strength and hope.

- Jake, recovering from surgery, told the Mayo Clinic Health System that focusing on gratitude before bed improved his sleep, which helped his healing.

Relaxation and Physical Activities to Support Healing

Relaxation and physical activity are vital in reducing Stress and supporting healing. Techniques like meditation, guided imagery, and physical exercise can help shift your mindset from anxiety to calm and improve your body's response to treatment.

Guided Meditation: Listening to a recorded guide can help you visualize a peaceful place, release tension, and cultivate positive feelings. Guided meditations are available on popular platforms like YouTube, Insight Timer, and many mobile apps.

Breathing Exercises: Techniques such as diaphragmatic breathing and the 4-7-8 technique can be used any time anxiety arises, helping to calm the nervous system and reduce overwhelming feelings.

You can combine breathing exercises with meditation and reenergize your energy by paying attention to the flow of energy in your breath. When you inhale, guide the breath slowly to the base of your spine, hold it there for 7 seconds, and breathe out slowly, guiding it wherever you feel it needs re-energizing.

Visualization involves imagining a positive treatment outcome or visualizing that your body is successfully fighting cancer. Many survivors find this technique empowering, as it helps them focus on hope and healing.

Physical Activity for Well-being

Yoga and Stretching: Gentle yoga poses, such as child's pose and cat-cow stretch, can relieve tension and boost mood. Yoga not only strengthens the body but also improves flexibility and relaxation.

Head massaging: Head massages can provide substantial relief and comfort for you by helping manage symptoms such as anxiety, fatigue, and tension. The gentle stimulation from head massages can improve circulation, which promotes relaxation, enhances mood, and reduces stress levels. This massage is especially beneficial for those dealing with the emotional and physical challenges of cancer treatment, as massages encourage the release of endorphins that alleviate discomfort and improve sleep quality.

You can perform a gentle self-massage on the scalp to reduce tension, alleviate Stress, and promote relaxation. Using the fingertips, you can start at the hairline and gently move in small, circular motions across the scalp, focusing on areas that often hold tension, such as the scalp, neck, and upper shoulders, applying light pressure to avoid irritation. This massage encourages blood flow, soothing the area and reducing fatigue. For added relaxation, you may find that using a small amount of natural oil, such as lavender or chamomile, can help calm the senses and enhance the overall experience.

This type of therapeutic touch, often part of a broader integrative care approach, can contribute significantly to overall well-being, enhancing both physical resilience and mental tranquility during cancer recovery.

Walking:

Walking is one of the simplest ways to stay active. A daily walk in a natural environment can improve mood, reduce anxiety, and boost energy. Many cancer survivors find strength and positivity in walking as part of their daily routine, contributing significantly to their mental and physical resilience during and after treatment. Here are a few inspiring stories:

Mary Pat Tiedemann, a stage 4 esophageal cancer survivor, walked daily along the Mississippi River to stay connected to her treatment journey and appreciate her second chance at life. Each walk became a personal ritual of gratitude and healing as she reflected on the support she received and the progress she made each day.

Kathy, a breast cancer survivor, used daily walks to help manage her mental health and physical strength during treatment. She was walking, which allowed her to connect with nature, which she described as grounding and energizing. This routine gave her a sense of accomplishment and control at a time when other aspects of her life felt uncertain.

CDC's Cancer Survivor Stories also highlight various survivors who incorporated walking as part of their post-treatment recovery, using it to regain strength, clear their minds, and stay active, emphasizing how even small steps forward can make a substantial difference in resilience and overall well-being.

These stories illustrate how daily walks help cancer survivors find balance, manage Stress, and cultivate gratitude during challenging times. Walking is a gentle form of physical exercise and a mental reprieve, helping patients stay positive and connected to their healing journey.

Tai Chi: Tai chi combines slow, deliberate movements with deep breathing, making it a perfect exercise for maintaining balance, flexibility, and mental clarity during treatment. If you have yet to hear of Tai Chi, you can watch and learn about it on the YouTube platform. If you are interested, you can join a Tai Chi group in your neighborhood. It is a good way to make new friends, too.

Building a Daily Practice

Building a daily practice of stress-reduction techniques can be simple and incredibly beneficial. Here are some exercises and tips:

Morning Meditation: Start each day with 10 minutes of guided meditation or prayer. Apps like Headspace and Calm offer free and easy-to-use resources to help you get started.

Morning affirmation: Repeating your favorite affirmations before engaging in your daily activities can help you feel confident with no fear.

Daily Breathing Exercises: Set aside 5 minutes daily for deep breathing. The 4-7-8 breathing exercise involves inhaling for 4 seconds, holding for 7 seconds, and exhaling for 8 seconds, which helps to relax your body and mind. Deep breathing is a powerful and easy-to-do tool you can use anytime, anywhere, when you feel anxious, upset, or stressed. It is best to do it first upon waking up and every two hours during the day.

Plan daily activities: Schedule time for stretching, head massaging, walking, and other activities like sports or gardening each day.

Evening Gratitude Practice: Write down three things you are grateful for and say them aloud each night. Practicing gratitude helps shift your focus from fear and Stress to positivity and hope.

In summary, the fight against cancer is not just physical—it is also emotional and mental. By cultivating hope, confidence, and resilience, you can positively impact your treatment journey and enhance your quality of life. Relaxation techniques, meditation, gentle exercise, and stress management are powerful tools that can help support your body and mind during this challenging time. Remember, you can shape your mindset and make choices that contribute to your healing journey.

References:

1. National Cancer Institute (NCI). (2022). Mind-Body Therapies in Cancer Treatment. Retrieved from https://www.cancer.gov/about-cancer/treatment/cam/mind-body

2. American Cancer Society. (2021). Mind-Body Practices for Cancer Patients. Retrieved from https://www.cancer.org

3. Memorial Sloan Kettering Cancer Center (MSKCC). Integrative Medicine: Mind-Body Therapies. Retrieved from https://www.mskcc.org/cancer-care/integrative-medicine

4. Bauer-Wu, S. (2010). Mindfulness Meditation and Cancer: Benefits for Cancer Patients and Survivors. Oncology Nursing Forum, 37(3), 234-240.

5. World Health Organization (WHO). (2022). Mental Health and Cancer Care: The Importance of Mind-Body Healing. Retrieved from https://www.who.int/mental-health

Chapter 10

Step-by-Step Guide to combining natural and standard therapies

A holistic approach can bring better results—learn how to integrate therapies for maximum benefit.

Combining natural and conventional therapies for cancer treatment can offer a comprehensive approach to healing. This chapter provides a step-by-step guide to navigating the journey of combining natural therapies with standard cancer treatments. From early detection to becoming a victor in the fight against cancer, we offer practical advice and real-life examples to help you achieve the best possible outcomes.

To effectively combine natural and conventional therapies, it is crucial to follow a structured approach. Here is a guide on how to do so:

Step 1: Check Your Health for Early Symptoms

If you have been diagnosed with cancer, skip steps 1 and 2 and go to step 3.

The first step is to assess your health to determine if you have any concerning symptoms. Make a complete list of the symptoms you have. Compare these symptoms with the early signs of different types of cancer below (from Chapter 4) to get a good idea of what types of cancer they may signal. Early detection is crucial, as it allows for more effective treatment.

Here are the early signs of the most common types of cancer

Breast cancer

- Lump or thickening in the breast or underarm.- Changes in breast shape or size. – Nipple discharge, especially if it's bloody.- Redness or dimpling of the skin on the breast (like an orange peel).- Inverted nipple or changes in the nipple's appearance.

Brain Cancer

- Headaches that become more frequent or severe.- Seizures.- Nausea or vomiting.- Vision problems (blurred vision, double vision).- Difficulty with balance or speech.- Changes in personality or behavior.- Weakness or numbness in one side of the body.

Skin cancer

- Changes in moles (size, shape, color, or texture).- New skin growths or sores that do not heal.- Itching, tenderness, or pain around a mole or spot.- Dark streaks under nails.- Unexplained bleeding from a mole.

Pancreatic cancer

- Jaundice (yellowing of the skin and eyes).- Dark urine and pale stools.- Abdominal or back pain that may radiate to the back.- Unexplained weight loss.- Loss of appetite.- New onset of diabetes (rising blood sugar level) or worsening of existing diabetes.

Gastric cancer

- Indigestion or persistent heartburn- Feeling bloated after eating, even a small meal.- Nausea or vomiting (sometimes with blood).- Unexplained weight loss. – Abdominal pain, especially after eating.

Liver cancer

- Unexplained weight loss.- Loss of appetite or feeling full quickly.- Abdominal pain or swelling, especially in the upper right quadrant.- Yellowing of the skin and eyes (jaundice).- Nausea and vomiting.- General fatigue and weakness.

Colorectal (Colon and Rectal) Cancer

- Changes in bowel habits, such as diarrhea, constipation, or narrowing of the stool.- Blood in the stool (either bright red or very dark). – Abdominal discomfort (cramping, pain, or bloating). – Unexplained weight loss.- Fatigue or weakness.

Prostate cancer

- Difficulty urinating (weak stream, frequent urination, especially at night).- Pain or burning sensation during urination. -Blood in the urine or semen.- Erectile dysfunction.- Pain in the hips, back, or pelvis (may indicate cancer has spread).

Lung cancer

- Chronic cough or a cough that worsens over time.- Coughing up blood (hemoptysis).- Shortness of breath or wheezing.- Chest pain that may worsen with deep breathing or coughing. – Hoarseness or voice changes.- Frequent respiratory infections, like bronchitis or pneumonia.

Oral Cancer

- Persistent mouth sores- White or red patches on the gums, tongue, or lining of the mouth- Lumps or thickening in the cheek or tongue may feel different from surrounding tissue.- Difficulty chewing or swallowing

Throat (Pharyngeal) and voice box (Laryngeal) Cancer

- Persistent sore throat, especially if other symptoms accompany it- Voice changes with hoarseness or unusual voice quality lasting more than two weeks – Difficulty swallowing with a feeling of food getting stuck or a sensation of something in the throat – Chronic cough with a cough that persists and isn't due to a cold or infection

Nasal and Sinus Cancers

- Persistent Nasal congestion or blockage, usually on one side only. – Frequent nosebleeds without any apparent cause – Facial pain or numbness: often around the eyes or upper teeth -Changes in the sense of smell

Neck and Head cancers:

- Swelling or lump in the neck: Painless swelling or lump, often in the lymph nodes, does not go away. -Unexplained significant weight loss without changes in diet or exercise – Ear pain or fullness: Persistent ear pain or a feeling of fullness, primarily if not related to ear infections.

Cervical Cancer

- Unusual vaginal bleeding. – Watery bloody discharge -Pelvic pain -Pain during urination

Ovarian Cancer

- Bloating -Pelvic or Abdominal Pain -Feeling Full Quickly -Frequent urination – Changes in bowel habits -Fatigue

Step 2: Make an appointment with Your Doctor for a Diagnosis and treatment plan

If cancer is suspected, make an appointment with your healthcare provider immediately for a formal diagnosis and treatment plan. To prepare for the appointment, read the diagnosis process relating to the suspected cancer in Chapter 2 to get a good idea about the coming diagnosis process.

Talk openly with your doctor about the symptoms you have been experiencing and what type of cancer you think they may relate to. Discuss with your doctor the expected diagnosis process. Make your doctor aware of your interest in combining natural therapies with conventional treatments and your plan to use some natural products while waiting for diagnosis and a conventional treatment plan. A collaborative approach from the outset is key to creating an effective treatment plan that combines the best of both worlds.

Step 3: Select the natural products most suitable for you and how to use them

After identifying the early symptoms and the type of cancer you have or may have, **go back to Chapter 7 and read** the suggested combined therapies for the related cancer.

Go through them carefully and **select** the natural products we want to use while waiting for the diagnosis based on their accessibility and affordability. You don't have to use all of them, even though the more, the better if they are easily accessible and can be easily incorporated into your daily routine, especially ginger, garlic, probiotics, and blueberries.

Then, write down the ones you select.

Step 4: Prepare and Use the natural products you selected

If you are waiting for the diagnosis you can start preparing and using them.

If you have been diagnosed or are under treatment, do not use them before discussing with your oncologist about your intention to incorporate the selected natural products into the treatment plan.

At the same time, read Chapters 8 and 9 about the role of nutrition and body and mind. Carefully make a diet plan and other lifestyle changes you need to implement. Start the new diet plan and activities to overpower the cancer cells.

Step 5: Attend the diagnosis process

Skip this step if you are already under treatment.

If the diagnosis indicates that you have cancer, you can ask your doctor the following

- *How accurate are the diagnostic methods being used?*

- *What stage is my cancer, and what does that mean for my treatment options?*

- *Should I get a second opinion?*

- *Are there any additional screenings or follow-up tests needed?*

Step 6: Understanding Your Treatment Options

- *If the diagnosis is negative, it is great news, but keep using the natural products until the symptoms go away. All* of them have therapeutic properties that address the symptoms at the root cause and restore your health.

- If the diagnosis is positive or you are already under treatment, you know the stage of cancer you are in. Go back to chapter 7 to see if a combined treatment plan for your case is among those suggested. If there is, please go through it carefully. If not, it is beneficial to read the section relating to the diagnosed cancer in Chapter 4 to educate yourself about your conventional treatment options, including chemotherapy, radiation, surgery, immunotherapy, and targeted therapies for the stage you are in. Gain a clear understanding of how these treatments work and the corresponding effectiveness of the conventional treatment.

Step 7: Get an agreed treatment plan for you with the oncologist.

After the diagnosis, the healthcare team will direct you to an oncologist or a team of oncologists. They will tell you their treatment plan, but they will probably not explain in detail what cancer drugs will be used.

- Go through with them the therapies that they want to use for you, whether Surgery, chemotherapy, radiotherapy, targeted therapy, hormone therapy and immunotherapy will be carried out. If your type of cancer is among the suggested combined therapies in chapter 7 and you want to follow the suggested combined therapies, it is time to let them know and discuss with them about the suggested combination.

- Go through the lists of drugs to be used or may be used.

- If the cancer you face is not among the common types that have suggested combined therapies in chapter 7, check if there are any drugs in the plan that may have unwanted interactions with your chosen natural products as listed in chapter 6. Briefly stop using those natural products that may have unwanted interactions with those drugs from 2 days before to 2 days after the drugs being administered. Remember that for each of specific cancer drug, there are still quite a few of natural products that can used to enhance the treatment and minimize its adverse effects. For example with *Doxorubicin:* we should avoid *Aloe Arborescens, Black cumin, Fucoidan, Garlic, Ginger, Papaya, Turmeric, Virgin Coconut Oil.* But we can use Bitter melon, Flaxseeds, Blueberries, Mistletoes, Perilla, Probiotics and Honey. (Chapter 6). With drugs that are similar to Doxorubicin, we do the same. (Look up Table 2 again)

- Convince the oncologist that you want to use natural products to enhance the effectiveness of conventional treatment while at the same time minimizing its adverse effects (as presented in Chapter 6). Discuss openly with your oncologists if they have any concern.

- You want to receive the best treatment results with a synergistic and complementary combination of natural and conventional therapies. Avoiding or reducing the doses of heparin, warfarin, or aspirin may resolve any concern about the additive blood-thinning effect of natural products.

- This is the most appropriate time to tell them what natural products you have used or want to use during the treatment.

- If you are already under treatment, you should immediately tell them you want to add natural therapies to complement the conventional treatment.

- Present to them clearly in writing the products you want and how you will use them.

- And discuss openly with them any of their concerns and your concerns, especially about the need and the possibility of increasing the treatment efficacy and minimizing side effects with your selected natural products.

- This step aims to get **an agreed treatment plan** to combine natural and conventional therapies during treatment. This step is crucial if you are in an advanced cancer stage from III to IV, where the effectiveness of traditional therapy alone is low due to drug resistance and low drug sensitivity of cancer cells.

Step 8: Monitor Your Progress

- Monitoring your body's response to conventional and natural therapies as you progress in your treatment journey is essential.

- Keep a record of the progress of your health conditions

- Share the results and any concerns with your healthcare team. They may adjust your treatment plan based on how your body responds to the combined therapies, ensuring the best possible outcomes.

- Make sure your condition is regularly checked by the team responsible for your treatment.

Step 9: Maintaining an Integrative Approach

Integrating natural therapies into your treatment should be an ongoing effort. Consider regular consultations with an oncologist or a healthcare provider with experience in natural therapies. This ongoing support will help you balance conventional and natural treatments, optimizing your overall well-being.

Step 10: Post-Treatment Care

After completing your conventional treatment, continue incorporating natural therapies to support recovery and prevent recurrence. Therapies such as meditation, nutritional supplements, and herbal products can help boost your immune system and reduce long-term side effects. Regular follow-up appointments with your healthcare team are crucial to monitor your progress and adjust your care plan as needed.

Consultation Tips

To communicate effectively with your healthcare team about natural therapies, consider the following:

- ***Be Honest and Open***: Share all details about any herbs, supplements, or natural products you are taking or considering. Transparency helps your healthcare provider give you the best advice.

- ***Monitor and Report:*** After starting a natural product, track any new symptoms or side effects and report them to your healthcare provider as soon as possible.

Conclusion

Combining natural and conventional therapies can offer a well-rounded and practical approach to cancer treatment. Following a step-by-step plan, working closely with healthcare providers, and making informed choices can enhance treatment outcomes while minimizing side effects. Remember, the key to successful integration is open communication and collaboration with your healthcare team, ensuring that you and your loved ones receive the best of both worlds for your and your loved ones' health and well-being.

Conclusion

Summarize, inspire, and empower—your journey toward better health is just beginning.

This book aims to empower you with the knowledge and confidence to make informed choices that support optimal healing. The emphasis remains on the value of combining conventional treatments with natural therapies to optimize healing and enhance quality of life. We hope this guide has shown you that you are not alone and can actively participate in your treatment. By embracing a balanced approach grounded in evidence-based medicine and holistic care, you're setting yourself up for the best possible outcomes.

Key Takeaways

Each chapter has equipped you with insights and strategies for navigating cancer treatment with more control and less fear. Understanding cancer, identifying early signs, knowing treatment options, and integrating supportive therapies have all been covered to help you make informed decisions. Take time to read and understand any part that relates to your or your loved one's condition so that you can take an active role in discussing the treatment plan with your doctor and oncologist.

Reaffirmation of Empowerment

You have the power to actively participate in your treatment journey, making choices that resonate with your values and health goals. Knowledge is your ally, and your proactive approach can foster physical healing and mental resilience.

Encouragement for a Hopeful and Proactive Mindset

As you move forward, remember that hope and determination are as important as any treatment. This book aims to inspire confidence that your actions, thoughts, and choices all contribute to your and your loved one's healing journey.

Importance of Cancer Prevention

For those who are caring for loved ones with cancer or are interested readers looking to avoid cancer, it is crucial to understand the value of prevention. The natural anticancer products, healthy diet, body mind activities and lifestyle habits presented in this book can not only support cancer treatment but also help prevent cancer from developing in the first place. By adopting these practices, you can significantly lower your risk of cancer and enhance your overall well-being, leading to a healthier, more vibrant life.

Life After Treatment: Embracing Recovery and Resilience

Completing cancer treatment is a significant milestone, but for many, the journey doesn't end there. The lingering effects of conventional treatments—whether physical, emotional, or mental—can continue to impact daily life. This book is here to help you navigate this stage of healing by offering natural and practical strategies to alleviate side effects, rebuild your strength, and restore a sense of balance and well-being. It provides valuable guidance for both survivors and their carers, empowering you to manage challenges and focus on recovery together.

By adopting holistic practices such as nourishing your body with wholesome foods, engaging in restorative exercises, and embracing mind-body techniques like mindfulness or meditation, you can address lingering fatigue, pain, or emotional distress. For carers, this book also offers insights into supporting your loved one while maintaining your own well-being. Together, you can take positive steps toward a healthier, more vibrant life, letting go of the fear of recurrence and focusing on living fully in the present.

Request for Engagement and Community

Thank you for reading this book to the end. We love to hear about your experience with this book and its impact on your journey. Reviews are welcome and much appreciated, and for further support, we encourage you to connect with the author or join relevant support communities. Contact information and resources are available to help you stay connected and find the support you need. (To give a review on Kindle, please open (click on) the last page of the book, then swipe to open the next page, a review form will appear for you).

Final Message of Hope

This book is not the end of your journey—it's a foundation for a hopeful, informed, and empowered path forward. Every small step you take, every question you ask, and every decision you make are all part of your healing. Remember, cancer treatment is not just about targeting the disease; it's about nurturing the whole person.

Resources for Further Support:

Please refer to the resources section or reach out directly for continued guidance and community support. Many cancer organizations and support networks can provide additional assistance and a listening ear as you navigate this journey.

Contact Information: For questions, feedback, or to share your journey, you can contact the author through the following channels:

- **Email**: truwaynenz@gmail.com

- **Social Media**:
    - **Instagram**: @truwaynebooks

Feel free to connect for updates, additional resources, or simply to share your story.

Sources of Information:

1. American Cancer Society (ACS): This organization provides guidelines and detailed information on cancer treatments, treatment options, side effects, clinical trials, and survival rates. It also offers guidance on diet and nutrition during cancer treatment.

2. National Cancer Institute (NCI): This institute offers extensive resources on cancer therapy, effectiveness, clinical trials, and the effectiveness of treatments for various stages of cancer, including cancer statistics. It also provides resources on complementary and alternative therapies.

3. Mayo Clinic: Well-respected medical source with patient-centered information on cancer therapies, side effects, their effectiveness across different stages

4. Colorectal Cancer Alliance: A valuable resource for up-to-date information on therapies and survival statistics.

5. Lung Cancer Research Foundation (LCRF): This organization provides up-to-date information on advances in lung cancer therapies and clinical trials.

6. Hepatitis B Foundation: Information on liver cancer related to

hepatitis B, a common cause of liver cancer worldwide.

7. World Health Organization (WHO): Global Cancer Observatory (https://gco.iarc.fr/)

8. National Cancer Institute (NCI): SEER Cancer Statistics (https://seer.cancer.gov/)

9. National Institute of Health: Clinical studies and reviews on cancer treatments (https://pubmed.ncbi.nlm.nih.gov/)

10. Research Journals: Journal of Agricultural and Food Chemistry, Journal of Cancer Research and Clinical Oncology, Oxidative Medicine and Cellular Longevity, and Molecular Nutrition & Food Research.

11. Medical Databases: PubMed, ScienceDirect and Google Scholar provide access to peer-reviewed research on blueberries and cancer.

12. Institutional Resources: The National Cancer Institute (NCI) and Memorial Sloan Kettering Cancer Center offer information on the use of dietary supplements and foods in cancer care.

13. PubMed: To access studies on natural products in cancer treatment (search for terms with the product names and cancer, such as "ginger cancer" or "garlic cancer").

14. Memorial Sloan Kettering Cancer Center—About Herbs Database: This database provides evidence-based information on herbs and plant foods for cancer patients.

15. American Institute for Cancer Research (AICR): Discusses the role of diet and specific foods in cancer prevention and treatment.

16. ClinicalTrials.gov: Lists ongoing and completed clinical trials related to the use of different natural products in cancer treatment.

17. National Center for Biotechnology Information (NCBI): Provides peer-reviewed studies on the effects of mistletoe on cancer cells, including its immune-boosting and apoptotic properties. https://www.ncbi.nlm.nih.gov

18. Journal of Integrative Cancer Therapies: This journal publishes research on mistletoe extract's impact on immune function and tumor growth, as well as patient-reported outcomes.

19. Supportive Care in Cancer: Features studies highlighting mistletoe's role in improving quality of life and reducing chemotherapy side effects. https://link.springer.com/journal .

20. European Journal of Cancer: This journal includes research and reviews on the use of mistletoe extract as a complementary treatment in oncology, detailing its mechanisms of action and clinical benefits.

Appendix 1

Natural Allies: Powerful Plant-Based Therapies for Cancer

Explore nature's arsenal—plant-based therapies that can support cancer treatment with fewer side effects.

Nature offers a treasure trove of resources that can complement conventional cancer treatments, helping to ease side effects and boost overall well-being. For those navigating the challenges of cancer, plant-based therapies present an opportunity to draw on the healing powers of nature to support the body, mind, and spirit. While current conventional therapies struggle to completely eradicate cancer stem cells (CSC) because these cells often possess robust DNA repair mechanisms, enabling them to survive traditional treatments and even adapt to evade them, thus reducing the efficacy of treatment, research has found that some natural products such as , black cumin and perilla that can kill or inhibit the survival of CSC.

These appendices will present well-researched natural therapies that have shown potential in supporting cancer treatment, specifically Aloe arborescent, bitter melon, black cumin, flaxseeds, fucoidan, garlic, ginger, mistletoe, papaya, perilla, probiotics, turmeric, and virgin coconut oil. These natural therapies are backed by growing scientific evidence and centuries of traditional use, balancing modern and ancient wisdom. By understanding how each of these natural allies works, we can make informed decisions that complement conventional therapies, reduce adverse effects, and improve quality of life. We will also explore practical ways to integrate these therapies into daily routines, ensuring a comprehensive approach to cancer care that is both effective and manageable.

Summary

1. **Natural Therapies Overview**: These appendices introduces a range of natural therapies that have been researched for their ability to support cancer treatment. We explore their mechanisms of action, the health benefits they provide, and potential interactions with conventional medicines. Each therapy is chosen for its proven effects and its promise in alleviating side effects or enhancing the effectiveness of traditional cancer treatments.

2. **Evidence-Based Information**: The therapies discussed in these appendices are all supported by clinical studies or have compelling traditional uses supported by modern research. For each therapy, we will examine its specific properties and how they work in conjunction with cancer treatments. Understanding these mechanisms is crucial to safely and effectively incorporating them into your health regimen.

Aloe arborescens

Aloe arborescens is a perennial succulent plant from the Aloe genus, closely related to Aloe vera. It is native to southern Africa and has been used for centuries in traditional medicine in Africa and Asia for wound healing, skin conditions, and digestive issues. Recently, Aloe arborescens has gained attention for its potential therapeutic properties, particularly in alternative health practices. It has anti-inflammatory, antioxidant, immuno-modulatory, anti-cancer, laxative, digestive-enhancing, antibacterial, anti-fungal, skin healing, moisturizing, anti-aging, and detoxifying properties.

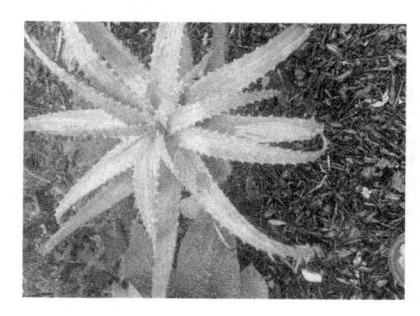

Aloe arborescens has been studied for its potential in cancer treatment and as a supportive therapy to enhance the effectiveness of standard cancer therapies such as chemotherapy and radiotherapy. Its properties can help neutralize the adverse effects of these treatments and improve the quality of life for cancer patients. Aloe arborescens show potential as a complementary therapy in cancer treatment, particularly for skin cancer, lung cancer, colon cancer, and liver cancer. Following are its potential benefits for cancer patients :

1. Enhancement of Chemotherapy and Radiotherapy Effectiveness

Synergistic Effects with Chemotherapy: Aloe arborescens contains bioactive compounds like aloin, aloe-emodin, and polysaccharides that can enhance the cytotoxic (cancer-killing) effects of chemotherapy. Studies suggest that these compounds help to inhibit cancer cell proliferation, induce apoptosis (programmed cell death), and increase the sensitivity of cancer cells to chemotherapy.

Radio-protective Effects: Aloe arborescens have radio-protective properties that can shield healthy cells from the damaging effects of radiation therapy. At the same time, it may enhance the radiosensitivity of cancer cells, making them more vulnerable to radiation, thus improving the overall efficacy of radiotherapy.

Inhibition of Cancer Cell Growth: Aloe arborescens has demonstrated the ability to inhibit cancer cell growth directly. Its compounds can interfere with the replication and division of cancer cells, slowing tumor progression and making other treatments more effective.

2. Protection against Chemotherapy and Radiotherapy Toxicity

Antioxidant Properties: Chemotherapy and radiation therapy generate oxidative stress, damaging healthy cells. Aloe arborescens contains high levels of antioxidants, including vitamins C and E, flavonoids, and carotenoids, which neutralize free radicals and protect cells from oxidative damage. These properties help reduce side effects like inflammation, tissue damage, and organ toxicity.

Detoxification: Aloe arborescens helps detoxify the body by promoting the elimination of toxins, which can build up during cancer treatment. This action supports liver and kidney function, which are often stressed by the toxic load of chemotherapy and radiotherapy.

3. Reduction of Chemotherapy and Radiotherapy Side Effects

Alleviation of Gastrointestinal Problems: Aloe arborescens is known for its soothing effects on the gastrointestinal tract. It can help relieve chemotherapy-induced nausea, vomiting, and digestive disturbances by healing the mucosal lining of the stomach and intestines. It also promotes bowel regularity, reducing the risk of constipation or diarrhea, which are common side effects of cancer treatment.

Prevention and Treatment of Mucositis: Oral and gastrointestinal mucositis (inflammation and ulcers) is a painful side effect of chemotherapy and radiation therapy. Aloe arborescens can soothe and heal mucous membranes, reducing the severity and duration of mucositis. Its anti-inflammatory and wound-healing properties help protect the mucosal tissue from further damage.

Skin Protection from Radiation Burns: Aloe arborescens can help heal skin wounds and burns. When applied topically, aloe gel can help prevent or treat radiation-induced skin burns, promoting faster healing and reducing pain, itching, and discomfort.

4. Immune System Support

Immuno-modulation: Aloe arborescens is rich in polysaccharides, particularly acemannan, which have immune-boosting properties. It can stimulate the immune system by enhancing the activity of macrophages, T-cells, and natural killer (NK) cells, which are critical in recognizing and destroying cancer cells. This immunomodulatory effect is essential, especially during chemotherapy, when chemo drugs often suppress the immune system.

Antimicrobial Properties: Cancer patients undergoing chemotherapy and radiotherapy are more susceptible to infections due to weakened immune systems. Aloe arborescens have natural antimicrobial properties, which can help prevent and treat infections, reducing the need for antibiotics and enhancing the body's natural defenses.

5. Anti-Inflammatory Effects

Reduction of Inflammation: Chronic inflammation is a hallmark of cancer progression and is often worsened by chemotherapy and radiotherapy. Aloe arborescens contain compounds like aloin and aloe-emodin that possess anti-inflammatory properties, which can reduce systemic inflammation. This property leads to decreased pain, swelling, and overall discomfort during treatment.

Support for Joints and Muscles: Many cancer patients experience joint and muscle pain as side effects of chemotherapy. Aloe's anti-inflammatory properties can help alleviate this pain, providing relief and improving mobility.

6. Pain Relief

Analgesic Properties: Aloe arborescens has mild analgesic effects, which can help reduce cancer-related pain and discomfort associated with chemotherapy and radiotherapy. Lowering inflammation and soothing damaged tissues help ease the pain, potentially reducing the need for strong painkillers.

7. Improvement in Quality of Life:

Enhanced Energy and Vitality: Chemotherapy often causes extreme fatigue and weakness. Aloe arborescens, with its detoxifying, anti-inflammatory, and immune-boosting properties, can help boost energy levels. It can also improve overall vitality, helping patients feel more energetic and better able to cope with treatment.

Better Nutrient Absorption: Cancer treatments can interfere with digestion and nutrient absorption. Aloe arborescens improves gut health and nutrient absorption, ensuring that cancer patients get the maximum benefit from their diet and supplements. This effect is critical for maintaining strength and body weight during treatment.

Mental Well-Being: Reducing pain, inflammation, and side effects, along with improving energy levels, can positively impact the mental health and emotional well-being of cancer patients. By alleviating physical symptoms, Aloe arborescens can help reduce anxiety, depression, and the overall psychological burden of cancer treatment.

8. Direct Anti-Cancer Properties

Induction of Apoptosis: Aloe arborescens can directly induce apoptosis, the process by which cancer cells self-destruct. This makes it a potential adjunct in cancer treatment, as it can target and kill cancer cells without harming healthy tissue.

Anti-Angiogenic Effects: The plant has shown its ability to inhibit angiogenesis, the process by which new blood vessels form to supply nutrients to tumors. By preventing angiogenesis, Aloe arborescens help starve tumors, slowing their growth and progression.

9. Improved Recovery and Healing

Faster Recovery Post-Treatment: Aloe arborescens' ability to support the immune system, reduce inflammation, and detoxify the body can help cancer patients recover more quickly from the damaging effects of chemotherapy and radiotherapy. Its regenerative properties promote faster healing of tissues damaged by cancer treatments.

Support for Emotional and Mental Resilience: Dealing with cancer can be detrimental to mental health. By reducing physical discomfort and promoting general well-being, Aloe arborescens can contribute to a better mental outlook and greater emotional resilience during the cancer journey.

Clinical Studies

Clinical studies have shown that Aloe arborescens can provide significant benefits for cancer patients, both in enhancing immune response and improving quality of life. A study published in the Journal of Cancer Research and Clinical Oncology found that Aloe arborescens extract, when used alongside chemotherapy, helped reduce the toxic side effects of the treatment while enhancing its effectiveness. The extract appeared to protect healthy cells from chemotherapy-induced damage and helped in reducing fatigue and other common side effects.

A clinical trial conducted by the National Center for Biotechnology Information (NCBI) demonstrated that Aloe arborescens extract helped improve immune function by increasing the activity of natural killer (NK) cells and T-lymphocytes, which are crucial for the body's ability to fight cancer. Patients using Aloe arborescens alongside their conventional treatments reported improved energy levels, better tolerance to chemotherapy, and an enhanced sense of well-being.

In the book "Cancer can be cured," the author recited how a lot of people had their cancer cured by using a Brazilian recipe of Aloe Arborescens juice with honey and some distillate. The types of cancer cured had a wide range from prostate to head and neck cancers. In the introduction, I also mentioned how Thora's father lived cancer-free for over 15 years until passing away after using this recipe alongside conventional treatment.

Patient Testimonials: Cancer patients who have used Aloe arborescens as part of their treatment plan reported positive outcomes, such as reduced nausea, improved digestion, and faster recovery times. Some patients have noted that applying the gel helped alleviate radiation burns and skin irritation while consuming aloe juice supported their immune function and overall vitality. Many have found Aloe arborescens a gentle yet effective addition to their cancer treatment, providing both physical relief and emotional support during a challenging time.

How to take Aloe Arborescens

Practical applications include consuming aloe juice or using aloe-based topical treatments to alleviate skin irritation caused by radiation. Aloe juice can be mixed with other juices to improve its taste, or it can be taken on its own to support digestion and enhance overall well-being. Topical application of aloe gel can also help soothe burns, reduce inflammation, and promote faster healing of the skin. Additionally, Aloe arborescens can be incorporated into smoothies or taken in supplement form, making it a versatile option for cancer patients looking to support their treatment and recovery.

Another aloe recipe for fighting cancer alone or with standard treatment is to mix the juice of 2 aloe arborescence leaves of 5 plus year old plants with half a kilo of raw honey and 3-4 tablespoons of distilled liquors (such as whiskey, tequila, vodka, or cognac). Normal dosage for cancer treatment is 1 table spoons three times a day between meals. This youtube video shows how to make the mix, called Zago's recipe: https://youtu.be/iZtBLFNbhJY?si=r6HyqqAF3qJ8pIYr

References:

1. Lissoni P., et al. (2009). A randomized study of chemotherapy versus biochemotherapy with chemotherapy plus Aloe arborescens in patients with metastatic cancer. In Vivo. 2009 Jan-Feb;23(1):171-5. PMID: 19368145. https://pubmed.ncbi.nlm.nih.gov/19368145/

2. Imanishi, K., et al. (2016). *Anticancer Effects of Aloe Arborescens on Human Cancer Cells.* Oncology Letters, 12(2), 1791-1797.

3. Kim, H. J., et al. (2015). *The Role of Aloe Arborescens Extracts in Enhancing Chemotherapy Efficacy.* Phytomedicine, 22(7-8), 715-723.

4. National Center for Biotechnology Information (NCBI). (2017). *Aloe Arborescens in Supportive Cancer Care.* Retrieved from https://www.ncbi.nlm.nih.gov

5. Aloe Arborescens and Cancer Treatment. (2021). *Complementary and Alternative Medicine Journal.* Retrieved from https://www.camjournal.org

Bitter Melon

Native to Asia and Africa, bitter melon (*Momordica charantia*) is a fruit commonly used in traditional Ayurvedic and Chinese medicine to manage blood sugar levels and to support digestive health. In recent times, it has been explored for anti-cancer potential.

It contains bioactive compounds like charantin, momordicoside, and polypeptide-p, which are believed to have anti-cancer properties. While studies on bitter melon's cancer-fighting potential are still in the early stages, preclinical research suggests it may be beneficial for certain types of cancer due to its ability to induce apoptosis (cell death), inhibit cell proliferation, and regulate blood sugar levels. These include breast, pancreatic, colon, liver, prostate, gastric, leukemia and skin cancers.

How Bitter Melon May Help Fight Cancer:

Induction of Apoptosis:

Bitter melon extract has been shown to trigger apoptosis, or programmed cell death, in cancer cells. This is essential for eliminating damaged or abnormal cells, a process often disrupted in cancer. Bitter melon may reduce tumor growth by restoring the normal cell death cycle.

Inhibition of Proliferation:

Bitter melon extract may inhibit the proliferation of cancer cells by targeting specific pathways that promote rapid and uncontrolled cell growth. Studies have shown that bitter melon affects proteins like mTOR and AMPK, which are involved in cancer cell metabolism and growth through cancer stem cells.

Antioxidants properties

Bitter melon has antioxidant properties that can help neutralize harmful free radicals. However, this effect may have a dual role in cancer treatment. While it protects healthy cells, it might also counteract specific cancer therapies that rely on oxidative stress to kill cancer cells (as seen with some chemotherapy drugs).

Regulation of Blood Sugar:

Bitter melon is widely known for its role in lowering blood sugar levels, which may be beneficial in cancers where insulin resistance and obesity are risk factors, such as breast, endometrial, and pancreatic cancer. Maintaining normal blood sugar levels is crucial for cancer patients, as elevated insulin can promote cancer growth.

Types of Cancer Bitter Melon May Help:

Research on bitter melon has shown potential efficacy in preclinical (lab and animal) models for several types of cancer:

Breast Cancer: Bitter melon extract has been studied for its ability to inhibit breast cancer cell proliferation. Studies suggest that it may disrupt pathways critical to the growth of breast cancer cells, such as the mTOR and Wnt signaling pathways.

Pancreatic Cancer: Research has demonstrated that bitter melon extract induces apoptosis in pancreatic cancer cells, reducing tumor growth in animal models. Pancreatic cancer cells are particularly sensitive to the blood sugar-lowering effects of bitter melon, which may contribute to its effectiveness. Research also demonstrated that bitter melon juice increases the sensitivity of pancreatic cancer stem cells to the chemotherapy drug gemcitabine, thus increasing its effectiveness.

Colon Cancer: Preclinical studies have shown that bitter melon inhibits the growth of colon cancer cells. Researchers suggest the regulation of inflammation and the induction of apoptosis as mechanisms for its anti-cancer effects in this context.

Lung Cancer: Bitter melon has demonstrated potential in reducing the proliferation of lung cancer cells by triggering apoptosis and interfering with cancer cell metabolism.

Prostate Cancer: Bitter melon extract may help inhibit prostate cancer cell growth by modulating pathways involved in cancer cell survival and death.

Clinical Studies

Clinical studies have shown that bitter melon can significantly benefit cancer patients, especially due to its anti-cancer and immune-boosting properties. A study published in the Journal of Ethnopharmacology demonstrated that bitter melon extract can inhibit the growth of cancer cells and induce apoptosis (programmed cell death) in various cancer types, including breast, prostate, and pancreatic cancers. The antioxidants found in bitter melon also help reduce oxidative stress, which benefits patients undergoing chemotherapy or radiation therapy.

A clinical trial conducted by the National Center for Biotechnology Information (NCBI) showed that bitter melon extract has immune-modulating effects. It enhances the activity of natural killer (NK) cells and boosts the body's ability to fight cancer. Patients who used bitter melon as part of their treatment plan reported better tolerance to chemotherapy, reduced inflammation, and improved energy levels.

Patient Testimonials:

Cancer patients who have incorporated bitter melon into their treatment plans reported positive outcomes, such as reduced treatment-related fatigue, better digestion, and enhanced immune function. Many patients have found that consuming bitter melon juice or supplements helped improve their overall well-being, with some reporting reduced pain and inflammation. Testimonials also highlight that bitter melon helped regulate blood sugar levels, which is particularly helpful for those at risk of treatment-related hyperglycemia.

References:

1. Panchal K, Nihalani B, Oza U, Panchal A, Shah B. Exploring the mechanism of action bitter melon in the treatment of breast cancer by network pharmacology. *World J Exp Med* 2023; 13(5): 142-155 [PMID: 38173546 DOI: 10.5493/wjem.v13.i5.142]

2. Ray R.B., et al. (2010). Bitter melon (*Momordica charantia*) extract inhibits breast cancer cell proliferation by modulating cell cycle regulatory genes and promotes apoptosis. *Cancer Res.* 70, 1925–1931 (2010). [Abstract]

3. Methanolic Extracts of Bitter Melon Inhibit Colon Cancer Stem Cells by Affecting Energy Homeostasis and Autophagy. https://onlinelibrary.wiley.com/journal/4747

4. Li, C.J., et al. (2012). Momordica charantia Extract Induces Apoptosis in Human Cancer Cells through Caspase- and Mito-

chondria-Dependent Pathways. Evid Based Complement Alternat Med. 2012;2012:261971. doi: 10.1155/2012/261971. Epub 2012 Oct 4. PMID: 23091557; PMCID: PMC3471438. https://pmc.ncbi.nlm.nih.gov/articles/PMC3471438/

5. Sur, S., Ray, R.B. (2020). Bitter Melon (*Momordica Charantia*), a Nutraceutical Approach for Cancer Prevention and Therapy. Cancers (Basel). 2020 Jul 27;12(8):2064. doi: 10.3390/cancers12082064. PMID: 32726914; PMCID: PMC7464160. https://pmc.ncbi.nlm.nih.gov/articles/PMC7464160/

Black Cumin *(Nigella Sativa)*

Black cumin seeds, or "black seed," have been used for thousands of years across the Middle East and Asia for their healing properties. Known as a remedy for "everything but death," these seeds have been valued for their potential in immune support, respiratory health, and digestive wellness.

Black cumin (Nigella sativa), particularly its active compound thymoquinone, has shown promise in enhancing the effectiveness of chemotherapy and alleviating its adverse effects for several types of cancer, including breast, colon, prostate, lung, pancreatic, and liver cancers. Black cumin seed oil and seeds are available at most Indian grocery stores. Here's how black cumin can potentially support cancer therapy and improve the quality of life for cancer patients:

1. Enhancement of Chemotherapy Effectiveness

Synergistic Effects with Chemotherapy: Studies suggest that black cumin and its active components (like thymoquinone) may work synergistically with chemotherapy drugs, increasing their effectiveness. For instance, thymoquinone has been found to enhance the sensitivity of cancer cells to chemotherapeutic agents, making cancer cells more susceptible to treatment.

Induction of Apoptosis *(Cancer Cell Death)*: Black cumin has induced apoptosis (programmed cell death) in cancer cells. Thymoquinone can inhibit cancer cell proliferation and promote the death of cancerous cells, thereby enhancing the anti-tumor effects of chemotherapy drugs.

Inhibition of Tumor Growth and Metastasis: Black cumin exhibits anti-tumor and anti-metastatic properties, helping slow cancer cell spread. This ability could potentially reduce the aggressiveness of tumors, complement chemotherapy, and improve patient outcomes. This effect may relate to thymoquinone's ability to inhibit the survival of cancer stem cells.

2. Protection against Chemotherapy-Induced Toxicity

Antioxidant Properties: Chemotherapy often leads to the production of reactive oxygen species (ROS), which can cause oxidative stress and damage healthy cells. Black cumin has potent antioxidant properties, which may help protect healthy cells from chemotherapy-induced oxidative damage. This antioxidant effect can reduce side effects such as fatigue, inflammation, and organ toxicity.

Organ Protection: Studies suggest that black cumin may protect organs like the liver, kidneys, and heart, which are often adversely affected by chemotherapy. Thymoquinone has reduced the toxicity of certain chemotherapeutic drugs, helping preserve the function of these critical organs during cancer treatment.

3. Reduction of Chemotherapy Side Effects

Alleviation of Gastrointestinal Issues: Chemotherapy can cause gastrointestinal problems, including nausea, vomiting, and loss of appetite. Black cumin has been used traditionally to soothe digestive issues, and its anti-inflammatory and antioxidant effects may help reduce chemotherapy-induced nausea and gastrointestinal discomfort.

Prevention of Hair Loss: Some studies suggest that black cumin oil may help mitigate hair loss caused by chemotherapy due to its nourishing and protective properties for hair follicles. However, more research is needed to confirm this.

Improved immune function: Chemotherapy often suppresses the immune system, leaving patients vulnerable to infections. Black cumin is known for its immune-boosting properties. Thymoquinone has been shown to modulate immune responses, potentially enhancing the body's ability to fight infections during chemotherapy.

4. Anti-Inflammatory Effects

Reduction of Inflammation: Black cumin's anti-inflammatory properties may help reduce the chronic inflammation often associated with cancer and chemotherapy. This effect can improve overall well-being and may reduce some of the systemic side effects of cancer treatment, such as pain and swelling.

5. Improvement in Quality of Life

Pain Relief: Thymoquinone, found in black cumin, has analgesic properties, which may help relieve cancer-related and treatment-related pain. This effect can improve the quality of life by reducing dependence on pain medications.

Enhanced Energy and Reduced Fatigue: The antioxidant effects of black cumin may help combat fatigue, a common side effect of chemotherapy. By reducing oxidative stress and inflammation, black cumin may improve energy levels and overall vitality.

Mood and Mental Health Support: Chemotherapy and cancer diagnosis can lead to anxiety and depression. Black cumin has been shown to have neuroprotective and mood-stabilizing properties, which may help improve mental health and emotional well-being in cancer patients.

6. Modulation of Cancer Cell Resistance

Overcoming Drug Resistance: One of the significant challenges in cancer treatment is the development of resistance to chemotherapy drugs. Black cumin, particularly thymoquinone, has been shown in some studies to reverse drug resistance in cancer cells, making them more susceptible to chemotherapy. This effect can enhance the long-term effectiveness of cancer treatment.

7. Support for Detoxification

Liver Support: The liver plays a crucial role in metabolizing chemotherapy drugs, and their toxicity can impair liver function. Black cumin has hepatoprotective properties, which can protect and support liver function during chemotherapy. This effect can enhance the body's ability to detoxify and process the drugs, reducing toxic buildup and side effects.

8. Anti-Cancer Properties of Black Cumin Alone

Direct Anti-Cancer Activity: Beyond its supportive role in chemotherapy, black cumin itself has been found to exhibit anti-cancer properties. Thymoquinone can inhibit cancer cell proliferation, block tumor growth, and even promote cancer cell death. This property suggests that black cumin could serve as a complementary therapy in cancer treatment.

Clinical Studies

Clinical studies have shown that black cumin seeds can significantly benefit cancer patients, particularly in boosting immunity and reducing tumor growth. A study published in the Journal of Cancer Research and Therapeutics found that thymoquinone, the active compound in black cumin seeds, has potent anti-cancer effects, including the induction of apoptosis (programmed cell death) in various cancer cells. The study demonstrated that black cumin seed extract could inhibit cancer cell proliferation and reduce tumor size, making it a promising complementary therapy.

A clinical trial conducted by the National Center for Biotechnology Information (NCBI) demonstrated that black cumin seed oil helped improve immune function in cancer patients by increasing the activity of natural killer (NK) cells and other immune components. Patients who used black cumin seed oil as part of their treatment plan reported better energy levels, reduced fatigue, and improved overall well-being.

A 2010 preclinical study reported in suggests that administration of NSO or TQ can lower cyclophosphamide (CTX) induced toxicity, as shown by an up-regulation of antioxidant mechanisms.

Evidence from preclinical studies reported in 2017 indicated that thymoquinone in black cumin can increase the effectiveness of conventional cancer treatments while protecting normal cells from therapy-associated toxic effects.

A retrospective clinical study reported in with 20 patients who had non-metastatic locally advanced inoperable pancreatic cancer revealed that consumption of black cumin oil and pure honey before and during chemoradiotherapy increased their survival time by 50%.

A study reported in found that consumption of black cumin containing thymoquinone before and following gemcitabine treatment caused increased apoptosis in pancreatic cancer cells and inhibited tumor growth.

Patient Testimonials:

Cancer patients who have incorporated black cumin seeds into their diet or treatment plan reported positive outcomes, such as reduced inflammation, improved immune function, and better tolerance to conventional treatments. Many patients have found that using black cumin oil in cooking or taking it as a supplement helped alleviate side effects like joint pain and digestive discomfort while also providing an energy boost. Testimonials also highlight the versatility of black cumin, with patients using it in both culinary and supplemental forms to support their overall health during cancer treatment.

References:

1. Khan A., Chen H., Tania M., Zhang D. (2011). Anticancer Activities of Nigella Sativa (Black Cumin) Afr J Tradit Complement Altern Med. 2011. https://www.sciencedirect.com/science/article/pii/S0975947616300389

2. Amin F. Majdalawieh, Muneera W. Fayyad (2016). Recent advances on the anti-cancer properties of *Nigella sativa*, a widely used food additive. Journal of Ayurveda and Integrative Medicine. https://www.sciencedirect.com/journal/journal-of-ayurveda-and-integrative-medicine/vol/7/issue/3

3. Alenzi, F.Q., El-Sayed El-Bolkiny, Y., M L Salem, M.L.(2010) Protective effects of Nigella sativa oil and thymoquinone against toxicity induced by the anticancer drug cyclophosphamide. https://pubmed.ncbi.nlm.nih.gov/20373678/

4. Tabish Mehraj, Rasha Mahmoud Elkanayati, Iqra Farooq, Tahir Maqbool Mir (2022). A review of *Nigella sativa* and its active principles as anticancer agents. https://www.sciencedirect.com/science/article/abs/pii/B9780128244623000123

5. Hannan, A., et al. (2021). Black Cumin (*Nigella sativa* L.) : A Comprehensive Review on Phytochemistry, Health Benefits, Molecular Pharmacology, and Safety. https://www.mdpi.com/2072-6643/13/6/1784

6. Kiziltan HS, Turkdogan MK, Gunes-Bayir A, et al. Can nigella sativa and pure honey improved chemoradiotherapy effects in advanced pancreatic cancer. *J Nutr Health Food Eng*. 2017;7(3):317-323. DOI: 10.15406/jnhfe.2017.07.00242

7. Tavakkoli, A., Mahdian, V., Razavi, B.M., Hosseinzadeh, H. (2017). Review on Clinical Trials of Black Seed (Nigella sativa) and Its Active Constituent, Thymoquinone. J Pharmacopuncture. 2017 Sep;20(3):179-193. doi: 10.3831/KPI.2017.20.021 . Epub 2017 Sep 30. PMID: 30087794; PMCID: PMC5633670.

8. Mostofa, A., et al. (2017) Thymoquinone as a Potential Adjuvant Therapy for Cancer Treatment: Evidence from Preclinical. Studies. https://www.frontiersin.org/journals/pharmacology/articles/10.3389/fphar.2017.00295/full

Blueberries

Blueberries have been used for centuries across various cultures for their health-promoting properties. Traditionally, Indigenous populations in North America valued blueberries not only as a nutritious food source but also for medicinal purposes.

Blueberries contain bioactive compounds, particularly anthocyanins and polyphenols that may offer benefits for cancer treatment as a complementary approach. Blueberries are available fresh, frozen, dried, juice, and powder. Here's a summary of how they can help cancer patients and common ways of taking them.

Antioxidant Properties: Blueberries are rich in antioxidants, which help neutralize free radicals, reducing oxidative stress that can contribute to cancer development.

Anti-inflammatory Effects: Chronic inflammation is associated with cancer progression. Blueberries contain compounds like quercetin and resveratrol that may help reduce inflammation.

Apoptosis and Cell Cycle Regulation: Blueberry polyphenols may encourage apoptosis (programmed cell death) in cancer cells and slow their proliferation, particularly in breast, colon, and prostate cancers.

Anti-metastatic Effects: Some compounds in blueberries can inhibit enzymes and signaling pathways involved in metastasis, potentially reducing cancer spread.

Chemotherapy Support: Blueberries may enhance the effects of chemotherapy. For example, they have been studied for their potential to improve response to treatments like doxorubicin in breast cancer.

Recommended Intake and How to Use Blueberries

Daily Serving: A typical recommendation is around 1/2 to 1 cup of fresh or frozen blueberries daily (about 75-150 grams). This amount can provide sufficient antioxidants and polyphenols for potential health benefits.

Forms to Use:

- Fresh or Frozen Berries: Ideal for preserving nutrients and bioactive compounds.

- Blueberry Powder or Extract: Concentrated forms can be used in smoothies or mixed into foods. Follow dosage instructions, typically around 1-2 teaspoons daily, but consult a healthcare provider for cancer-specific guidance.

- Blueberry Juice: Contains many beneficial compounds, though with reduced fiber. Limit intake to avoid excessive sugar.

References:

1. Johnson,S.A., Arjmandi, B.H. (2013). Evidence for anti-cancer properties of blueberries: a mini-review. Anticancer Agents Med Chem. 2013 Oct;13(8):1142-8. doi: 10.2174/18715206113139 990137. PMID: 23387969. https://pubmed.ncbi.nlm.nih.gov/23387969/

2. American Institute of Cancer Research (2021). Foods that fight cancer. Blueberries: Increase Antioxidant Activity in the Blood. https://www.aicr.org/cancer-prevention/food-facts/blueberries/

3. Ashique, S., et al. (2024). Blueberries in focus: Exploring the phytochemical potentials and therapeutic applications. https://www.sciencedirect.com/science/article/pii/S2666154324003375

4. Food for breast cancer (2024). Blueberries are highly recommended for breast cancer. https://foodforbreastcancer.com/foods/blueberries

Flaxseeds

Flax seeds (Linum usitatissimum), also known as linseeds, are small, golden, or brown seeds that have been cultivated for thousands of years for their nutritional and medicinal benefits. They originate from ancient Egypt and the Mediterranean.

They are known for their high content of omega-3 fatty acids, lignans, and fiber, which can offer multiple benefits in cancer prevention and treatment. These compounds have been studied for their potential to enhance the effectiveness of standard cancer therapies, reduce their adverse effects, and improve the quality of life for cancer patients.

Including flaxseeds in your diet can be as simple as adding ground flaxseed to smoothies, oatmeal, or baked goods, providing a versatile and nutritious boost. You can also mix flaxseed into yogurt, sprinkle it over salads, or use it as an egg substitute in baking by combining ground flaxseed with water. This way makes flaxseeds a nutritious addition and a functional ingredient that can enhance the texture and nutritional profile of your meals. Flaxseeds are usually available at supermarkets and food stores. Here are how flax seeds may help in cancer care:

1. Enhancement of Chemotherapy and Radiotherapy Effectiveness

Inhibiting the growth of hormone-related cancers: Flax seeds are one of the richest plant sources of lignans, a type of phytoestrogen. Lignans have been shown to have anticancer properties by inhibiting the growth of hormone-related cancers, particularly breast and prostate cancer. Lignans can bind to estrogen receptors and reduce the availability of active estrogen, which may slow the growth of estrogen-dependent cancer cells.

Inhibition of Tumor Growth: Lignans and omega-3 fatty acids found in flax seeds can inhibit tumor growth by blocking cancer cell proliferation and inducing apoptosis (cancer cell death). These compounds may enhance the effectiveness of chemotherapy by making cancer cells more vulnerable to treatment.

Anti-Angiogenesis Properties: Flax seeds contain bioactive compounds with anti-angiogenic effects. These compounds can prevent the formation of new blood vessels that tumors need to grow and metastasize. Flax seeds may also slow tumor progression and enhance the effectiveness of chemotherapy and radiotherapy by starving the tumor of nutrients and oxygen.

2. Protection against Chemotherapy and Radiotherapy Toxicity

Cell Protection: Flax seeds are rich in alpha-linolenic acid (ALA), a type of omega-3 fatty acid with anti-inflammatory properties. ALA can protect healthy cells from the oxidative damage caused by chemotherapy and radiotherapy while promoting the destruction of cancer cells. This protection may reduce the side effects of treatment, such as inflammation and tissue damage.

Antioxidant Support: Flax seeds' antioxidant properties, primarily through lignans and omega-3s, help neutralize free radicals generated during cancer treatments. This property can protect healthy cells and organs from damage, reducing side effects like nausea, fatigue, and organ toxicity (e.g., damage to the heart, liver, and kidneys).

3. Reduction of Chemotherapy and Radiotherapy Side Effects

Gastrointestinal Support: Flax seeds are high in fiber, which promotes healthy digestion and regular bowel movements. This is particularly beneficial for cancer patients undergoing chemotherapy, which can cause gastrointestinal side effects like constipation, diarrhea, and nausea. The mucilaginous fiber in flax seeds helps soothe the digestive tract, improving overall digestive health.

Prevention and Treatment of Inflammation: Chemotherapy and radiotherapy can cause inflammation in various body parts, including the gut, skin, and mucous membranes. Flax seeds, due to their high omega-3 content, have anti-inflammatory properties, which can help reduce inflammation and mitigate side effects like mucositis (inflammation of the mouth and digestive tract) and skin irritation from radiation therapy.

Reduction of Fatigue: Omega-3 fatty acids in flax seeds can help reduce chemotherapy-induced fatigue by lowering inflammation and supporting cellular repair processes. Improved energy levels can significantly enhance the quality of life for cancer patients during treatment.

4. Immune System Support

Immunomodulatory Effects: The lignans and omega-3 fatty acids in flax seeds have been shown to enhance immune function by modulating immune cell activity, reducing chronic inflammation, and supporting the body's natural defenses. A stronger immune system helps cancer patients better tolerate chemotherapy and recover more effectively between treatments.

Antimicrobial and Antiviral Properties: Flax seeds also contain bioactive compounds with antimicrobial and antiviral properties. This can help cancer patients, who are often immunocompromised due to chemotherapy, to better resist infections, thus improving their overall well-being and reducing complications.

5. Hormonal Regulation

Hormone-Dependent Cancer: Flax seeds are especially beneficial in hormone-related cancers like breast and prostate cancer. Lignans in flax seeds mimic estrogen in the body but in a weaker form, helping to regulate estrogen levels and inhibit the growth of hormone-dependent tumors. This property makes flax seeds particularly effective as a complementary therapy in cancers driven by hormonal imbalances.

6. Anti-Inflammatory Effects:

Systemic Inflammation Reduction: Chronic inflammation can fuel cancer progression and exacerbate the side effects of cancer therapies. The omega-3 fatty acids in flax seeds help reduce systemic inflammation by lowering the production of pro-inflammatory cytokines. This can alleviate pain, swelling, and discomfort associated with both cancer and its treatments.

Reduction of Joint and Muscle Pain: Cancer patients often experience joint and muscle pain as a side effect of chemotherapy. Flax seeds' anti-inflammatory properties can help relieve this pain, improving mobility and overall comfort during treatment.

7. Heart and Vascular Protection

Cardioprotective *Properties:* Some chemotherapy drugs, particularly anthracyclines, can damage the heart. The omega-3s in flax seeds can help improve heart health by reducing inflammation, lowering blood pressure, and improving cholesterol levels. This property can protect cancer patients from the cardiovascular side effects of chemotherapy, particularly those with pre-existing heart conditions.

Support for Blood Health: Chemotherapy can affect blood cells, leading to anemia or low platelet counts. Flax seeds' nutrients, including iron and omega-3s, can help support healthy blood production, potentially reducing the severity of chemotherapy-induced anemia and improving overall stamina.

8. Improvement in Quality of Life

Mood and Cognitive Support: Chemotherapy can lead to cognitive issues, often referred to as "chemo brain," as well as mood disturbances like depression and anxiety. The omega-3 fatty acids in flax seeds have neuroprotective properties that can help protect the brain from the cognitive side effects of chemotherapy and improve mood by supporting brain function.

Enhanced Energy and Well-Being: Flax seeds contain antioxidants, anti-inflammatory compounds, and essential fatty acids that can boost energy levels and reduce cancer-related fatigue. This effect contributes to improved well-being and a better ability to cope with cancer treatment.

9. Direct Anticancer Properties

Apoptosis Induction: Flax seeds can induce apoptosis in cancer cells, helping to promote the death of malignant cells. This effect, particularly in hormone-related cancers such as breast and prostate cancers, may slow the progression of the disease and improve patient outcomes when used alongside conventional therapies.

Anti-Metastatic Properties: Flax seeds may inhibit cancer metastasis by reducing inflammation, oxidative stress, and angiogenesis (the formation of new blood vessels that supply tumors). This effect may help limit the spread of cancer and improve survival rates in patients undergoing treatment.

10. Support for Detoxification

Liver Health: The liver is a crucial organ for detoxifying the body, especially during chemotherapy, when it has to process and eliminate toxic substances. Flax seeds contain nutrients that support liver health and promote detoxification, helping the body to remove toxins more efficiently and reduce chemotherapy-induced liver damage.

Improved Elimination of Toxins: Flax seed fiber aids in the elimination of toxins from the digestive tract, preventing their reabsorption into the bloodstream. This effect can reduce the overall toxic load on the body, easing the burden on detoxifying organs like the liver and kidneys.

Clinical Studies

Clinical studies have shown that flaxseeds can provide significant benefits for cancer patients, particularly those with hormone-related cancers. A study published in the Journal of Clinical Oncology found that the lignans in flaxseeds can help modulate hormone levels, which is beneficial for breast or prostate cancer patients. Flaxseeds have also been shown to slow tumor growth and reduce the risk of cancer recurrence due to their estrogen-modulating properties.

A clinical trial by the National Center for Biotechnology Information (NCBI) demonstrated that cancer patients who consumed flaxseeds experienced reduced inflammation, better hormonal balance, and improved overall prognosis. Flaxseeds' high fiber content also helped alleviate constipation, a common side effect of chemotherapy, thereby improving patients' digestive health.

Patient Testimonials:

Cancer patients who have incorporated flaxseeds into their diet reported positive outcomes, such as reduced fatigue, improved digestive health, and fewer hormone-related symptoms. Many patients have found that adding ground flaxseeds to smoothies or oatmeal helped them maintain energy levels and manage treatment side effects more effectively. Testimonials also highlight the versatility of flaxseeds, with patients using them in various recipes to easily integrate this powerful natural therapy into their daily routines.

References:

1. Merkher, Y., et al. (2023) Anti-Cancer Properties of Flaxseed Proteome. https://pmc.ncbi.nlm.nih.gov/articles/PMC10661269/

2. Calado, A., Neves, P.M., Santos, T., Ravasco, P. (2018) The Effect of Flaxseed in Breast Cancer: A Literature Review. https://pmc.ncbi.nlm.nih.gov/articles/PMC5808339/

3. Nowak, W., Jeziorek, M. (2023) The Role of Flaxseed in Improving Human Health. https://pmc.ncbi.nlm.nih.gov/articles/PMC9914786/

4. Thompson, L. U., et al. (2005). *Flaxseed and Its Lignans: Anti-*

cancer Properties and Mechanisms of Action. Journal of Nutrition, 135(5), 1207-1212.

5. Chen, J., & Saggar, J. K. (2007). *Flaxseed Components Reduce the Growth of Established Human Breast Tumors (MCF-7) in Mice.* Clinical Cancer Research, 13(3), 1061-1067.

6. National Center for Complementary and Integrative Health (NCCIH). (2022). *Flaxseed: Health Benefits and Cancer Research.* Retrieved from https://nccih.nih.gov

7. American Institute for Cancer Research (AICR). (2021). *The Role of Flaxseed in Cancer Prevention and Care.* Retrieved from https://www.aicr.org.

8. Buck, K., et al. (2011). *Dietary Intakes of Flaxseed and Flaxseed Components and Their Effects on Cancer Prognosis.* Nutrition and Cancer, 63(8), 1345-1353.

Fucoidan

Fucoidan is obtained from brown seaweeds like wakame and kombu and has been traditionally used in Japan and Korea for general wellness and longevity. Known for its potential immune-modulating and anti-inflammatory properties, it has been gaining attention in recent years for its potential benefits in cancer treatment. It's also being studied for its possible role in cancer support. Fucoidan possesses various biological activities, including anticancer, anti-inflammatory, and immune-boosting properties, which make it a promising complementary therapy for cancer patients. Fucoidan is mainly available in extract form from health shops and online. Following are how Fucoidan can help cancer patients:

Anticancer Properties: Fucoidan can induce apoptosis (programmed cell death) in cancer cells, a critical mechanism for controlling tumor growth. It also inhibits angiogenesis, in which tumors create new blood vessels to support their growth. By restricting blood flow to tumors, Fucoidan helps starve cancer cells of essential nutrients, hindering their progression.

Immune System Support: Fucoidan has immune-modulating effects that can enhance the activity of immune cells, such as natural killer (NK) cells and T cells, which are crucial for identifying and attacking cancer cells. This effect can help the body target and eliminate cancer cells more effectively, especially during conventional treatments that may weaken the immune system.

Reducing Side Effects of Chemotherapy: Chemotherapy can lead to various side effects, such as gastrointestinal discomfort and immune suppression. Fucoidan can protect healthy cells from chemotherapy's toxic effects while enhancing the treatment's efficacy. It can also help alleviate symptoms like nausea and inflammation, making the treatment more tolerable.

Inhibiting Cancer Metastasis: Fucoidan can inhibit cancer metastasis, which is the spread of cancer cells to other parts of the body. It works by interfering with molecules involved in cell adhesion and migration, which helps prevent the spread of cancer to distant organs.

Anti-Inflammatory Effects:

Chronic inflammation is associated with cancer progression. Fucoidan's anti-inflammatory properties help reduce inflammation, which may prevent cancer from advancing and support overall health during treatment.

Clinical Evidence:

1. Preclinical Studies: Laboratory studies have shown that Fucoidan can inhibit the growth of several cancer cells, including breast, lung, liver, and colon cancers. It can also enhance the effectiveness of chemotherapy drugs such as cisplatin, making it a valuable addition to conventional cancer therapies.

2. Clinical Trials: Some clinical trials have indicated that fucoidan supplementation can improve the quality of life for cancer patients. Participants reported reduced fatigue, improved immune function, and fewer side effects from chemotherapy. Fucoidan can improve tumor response to treatment, suggesting that it can act as a supportive therapy alongside conventional cancer treatments.

3. Patient Testimonials: Cancer patients who have used Fucoidan as a complementary therapy reported improved energy levels, reduced treatment side effects, and enhanced overall well-being. While individual experiences may vary, many patients find Fucoidan a beneficial addition to their cancer care regimen.

One concern with fucoidan supplements is that their composition can vary significantly depending on the source (seaweed species), extraction method, and formulation. This variability can affect efficacy and safety.

References:

1. Cao, L., et al. (2023) Antitumor activity of fucoidan: a systematic review and meta-analysis. https://pubmed.ncbi.nlm.nih.gov/35116386/

2. Lin, Y., et al. (2020) The anti-cancer effects of fucoidan: a review of both in vivo and in vitro investigations. Cancer Cell International. https://cancerci.biomedcentral.com/articles/10.1186/s12935-020-01233-8

Garlic

Garlic (Allium sativum) has been a folk medicine in ancient Egypt, Greece, and China for its potent medicinal properties. With its antibacterial, antiviral, and antifungal effects, garlic has traditionally been used to support heart health, enhance immunity, and combat infections. Studies have been carried out for their potential benefits in cancer prevention and as complementary therapies in cancer treatment

Below is an overview of the potential benefits of garlic for cancer patients, supported by clinical evidence and patient testimonials.

Immune System Support: Garlic has immune-boosting properties, which can benefit cancer patients, especially those undergoing treatments that suppress the immune system (e.g., chemotherapy or radiation).

A study published in the Journal of Nutrition (2001) found that aged garlic extract could enhance immune function, including increasing the activity of natural killer (NK) cells, which play a role in targeting and destroying cancer cells.

Anticancer Properties: Garlic contains sulfur compounds, such as allicin, diallyl disulfide (DADS), and Allyl Cysteine (SAC), which have demonstrated anticancer properties in laboratory and animal studies. These compounds work through multiple mechanisms, including promoting apoptosis, inhibiting cancer cell proliferation, and modulating cell signaling pathways involved in tumor growth.

Although large-scale clinical trials are limited, some studies suggest a correlation between garlic consumption and a reduced risk of certain cancers.

A meta-analysis published in the American Journal of Clinical Nutrition (2016) found that increased garlic consumption was associated with a reduced risk of several types of cancer, including colorectal, stomach, and prostate cancers.

A study in China (2006) found that regular consumption of garlic was associated with a 54% reduced risk of developing stomach cancer in people with high garlic intake compared to those with low intake.

Antioxidant and Anti-inflammatory Effects: Like ginger, garlic is rich in antioxidants that help fight oxidative stress, which contributes to cancer progression. Its anti-inflammatory properties may help reduce inflammation that can drive cancer development and complications from treatment.

A study published in Cancer Letters (2008) demonstrated that garlic extracts could inhibit the growth of breast cancer cells in vitro. The anticancer effects can downregulate specific pathways involved in cancer cell proliferation.

Cardiovascular Benefits: Cancer patients, mainly those undergoing treatment, may experience cardiovascular side effects. Garlic's cardiovascular benefits could help these patients by lowering blood pressure and improving cholesterol levels,

A study published in the International Journal of Preventive Medicine (2013) found that garlic supplementation improved cardiovascular health markers, including reducing blood pressure and cholesterol, which may be helpful for cancer patients at risk of cardiovascular complications due to treatment.

Detoxification and Chemoprotection: Garlic may help the body detoxify and remove harmful substances, including chemotherapy metabolites. This effect could potentially reduce the side effects of cancer treatment.

A 2010 study published in the European Journal of Cancer Prevention found that garlic could enhance the activity of liver enzymes involved in detoxification, suggesting that garlic might help reduce the toxic effects of chemotherapy.

Patient Testimonials

Some cancer patients report using garlic as a natural way to boost their immune system and improve their overall health during treatment. While not a substitute for conventional therapies, incorporating garlic into the diet becomes part of a holistic approach to care.

References:

1. Farhat, Z., et al. (2018). Types of garlic and their anticancer and antioxidant activity: a review of the epidemiologic and experimental evidence. European Journal of Nutrition. https://link.springer.com/article/10.1007/s00394-021-02482-7#

2. Thomson, M., Ali, M. (2003) Garlic [Allium sativum]: a review of its potential use as an anti-cancer agent. https://pubmed.ncbi.nlm.nih.gov/12570662/

3. Pandey, P., et al. (2023). Updates on the anticancer potential of garlic organosulfur compounds and their nanoformulations: Plant therapeutics in cancer management. https://www.frontiersin.org/journals/pharmacology/articles/10.3389/fphar.2023.1154034/full

Appendix 2

Natural Allies: Powerful Plant-Based Therapies for Cancer

Ginger

Ginger (Zingiber officinale) has been used in Ayurveda and traditional Chinese medicine for thousands of years. Known for its warming and anti-inflammatory properties, it is commonly used to aid digestion, relieve nausea, and alleviate joint pain. In recent decades, ginger has been studied for its potential benefits in cancer prevention and as a complementary therapy in cancer treatment. Here are the benefits of ginger for cancer patients:

Nausea and Vomiting Reduction (Especially in Chemotherapy): One of the most well-known uses of ginger is its ability to reduce nausea and vomiting, especially in patients undergoing chemotherapy.

Several studies have demonstrated ginger's efficacy in reducing chemotherapy-induced nausea and vomiting (CINV).

A 2012 study published in the Journal of Clinical Oncology found that ginger supplementation significantly reduced nausea severity in patients receiving chemotherapy. Patients who took ginger reported less severe nausea compared to those who took a placebo.

Another randomized controlled trial published in Supportive Care in Cancer(2017) confirmed ginger's anti-nausea effects, showing that it reduced nausea in breast cancer patients undergoing chemotherapy.

Anti-inflammatory and Antioxidant Effects: Ginger contains bioactive compounds like gingerol and shogaol, which have powerful anti-inflammatory and antioxidant effects. These properties are believed to help reduce chronic inflammation associated with cancer progression and improve the body's ability to fight oxidative stress, which may contribute to tumor development.

A study published in Cancer Prevention Research (2011) found that ginger extract could reduce markers of inflammation in the colon, suggesting potential benefits in reducing the risk of colon cancer. In the trial, participants who consumed ginger supplements significantly reduced pro-inflammatory markers in colon tissue, which may help reduce cancer risk or progression.

Pain Relief: Ginger can alleviate pain associated with cancer treatments, particularly when inflammation plays a role. A 2018 clinical trial involving women with breast cancer found that ginger supplementation helped reduce joint pain caused by aromatase inhibitors, drugs used in hormone-sensitive breast cancer treatment. This means ginger may be a valuable complementary treatment for pain management in cancer care.

Appetite Stimulation and Improved Digestion: Ginger may help improve appetite and promote better digestion, which can be affected by cancer and treatments like chemotherapy and radiation. Cancer patients often struggle with maintaining adequate nutrition due to treatment side effects, and ginger's ability to ease digestive discomfort can be beneficial.

Anticancer Properties (Preclinical Evidence): Ginger also shows potential as a direct anticancer agent in preclinical studies. Active compounds like 6-gingerol and 6-shogaol have inhibited the growth of various cancer cells in vitro and animal models.

Research published in PLoS One (2014) found that ginger extract induced apoptosis (programmed cell death) and inhibited proliferation in ovarian cancer cells.

Another study in The Prostate (2013) reported that ginger extract inhibited prostate cancer cell growth and progression in mice, suggesting that ginger may have potential as a preventive or complementary treatment.

Clinical evidence:

Cancer patients often report using ginger to alleviate chemotherapy-induced nausea and digestive issues. Many claim that it helps them tolerate their treatments better and improves their overall quality of life.

References:

1. Nachvak, S.M., et al (2022) Ginger as an anticolorectal cancer spice: A systematic review of in vitro to clinical evidence. Food Sci. Nutr. https://pubmed.ncbi.nlm.nih.gov/36789081/

2. Tôrres de Lima, R.M., et al. (2018) Protective and therapeutic potential of ginger (Zingiber officinale) extract and [6]-gingerol in cancer: A comprehensive review. https://pubmed.ncbi.nlm.nih.gov/30009484/

3. Aloqbi, A. A. (2024). Recent Updates on Unravelling the Therapeutic Potential of Ginger Bioactive Compounds in Cancer Man-

agement. *International Journal of Pharmaceutical Investigation*, *14*(3), 595–606. https://doi.org/10.5530/ijpi.14.3.72

4. Nerkar, A.G., Ghadge, H. (2022). Ethnopharmacological review of ginger for anticancer activity. DOI:10.18231/j.ctppc.2022.028 . https://www.researchgate.net/publication/365617918_Ethno pharmacological_review_of_ginger_for_anticancer_activity.

Honey

Honey has a long history across ancient civilizations like Egypt and Greece, where people used it as a natural sweetener and medicine. Known for its antibacterial, anti-inflammatory, and wound-healing properties, Honey is often used in traditional medicine to treat respiratory ailments, digestive issues, and skin infections.

Honey, mainly due to its rich antioxidant and anti-inflammatory properties, has been studied for its potential to enhance the effectiveness of chemotherapy, neutralize its adverse effects, and improve the overall quality of life for cancer patients. It is suitable as a complementary therapy for breast, colorectal, prostate, liver, skin, oral, head and neck, and gastrointestinal (gastric and esophageal) cancers. Here's how Honey can support cancer treatment:

1. Enhancement of Chemotherapy Effectiveness

Synergistic Effects with Chemotherapy: Honey, especially its phenolic compounds, may increase the sensitivity of cancer cells to chemotherapy, enhancing the treatment's efficacy. Some studies have suggested that Honey's bioactive components can work alongside chemotherapeutic agents to inhibit cancer cell growth more effectively than chemotherapy alone.

Inhibition of Tumor Growth: Honey exhibits direct anticancer properties, including the ability to inhibit the proliferation of cancer cells, induce apoptosis (programmed cell death), and inhibit tumor growth. This effect may complement chemotherapy by reducing the tumor's size or slowing its progression.

Prevention of Metastasis: Honey can help prevent cancer cells from metastasizing or spreading to other parts of the body. By reducing inflammation and affecting cell signaling pathways involved in cancer spread, Honey may act as a supportive therapy for chemotherapy.

2. Protection against Chemotherapy-Induced Toxicity

Antioxidant Protection: Chemotherapy often leads to generating reactive oxygen species (ROS), which causes oxidative stress and damage to both cancerous and healthy cells. Honey is a potent antioxidant, helping to neutralize ROS and protect healthy cells from oxidative damage. This effect can reduce chemotherapy-induced toxicity in vital organs like the heart, liver, and kidneys.

Organ Protection: Honey can protect against chemotherapy-induced organ damage. For instance, Honey can shield the liver, kidneys, and gastrointestinal system from the harmful side effects of specific chemotherapeutic agents. This protection helps maintain the function of these organs during treatment.

3. Reduction of Chemotherapy Side Effects

Reduction in Mucositis (Digestive tract inflammation): One of the most common side effects of chemotherapy is oral mucositis, which causes painful inflammation and ulceration in the mouth and digestive tract. Honey has demonstrated significant effectiveness in reducing the severity of mucositis in cancer patients undergoing chemotherapy or radiotherapy. Its soothing, anti-inflammatory, and wound-healing properties help to alleviate pain and promote faster healing of mucosal tissue.

Alleviation of Gastrointestinal Issues: Honey's anti-inflammatory and antioxidant properties can help reduce chemotherapy-induced gastrointestinal side effects such as nausea, vomiting, and diarrhea. It can help soothe the digestive system and promote a healthier gut environment.

Reduction in Fatigue: Chemotherapy-induced fatigue is a major challenge for cancer patients. Honey's energy-boosting and antioxidant properties may help reduce fatigue and improve overall vitality during cancer treatment.

4. Immune System Support

Enhanced Immune Function: Chemotherapy often weakens the immune system, leaving patients more susceptible to infections. Honey is known for its immune-boosting properties due to its antibacterial, antiviral, and antifungal effects. Regular consumption of Honey may help enhance immune function, reduce the risk of infections, and promote better recovery between chemotherapy cycles.

Wound Healing and Infections: Honey, particularly Manuka honey, has been used to treat wounds and infections. Its antibacterial properties can help prevent and treat infections common in immunocompromised cancer patients, particularly those receiving chemotherapy.

5. Anti-Inflammatory Effects

Reduction in Inflammation: Honey's anti-inflammatory properties can help reduce systemic inflammation caused by chemotherapy. This effect is beneficial not only in alleviating pain and swelling but also in reducing chronic inflammation that can fuel cancer progression. By lowering inflammation, Honey can improve comfort and overall well-being during treatment.

6. Pain Management

Analgesic Properties: Honey has natural pain-relieving properties that may help alleviate cancer-related pain and pain associated with chemotherapy side effects such as mucositis, digestive issues, and neuropathy (nerve pain). Its soothing effects may reduce the need for additional pain medications, improving quality of life.

7. Mood and Mental Health Support

Reduction in Anxiety and Depression: The high levels of antioxidants and anti-inflammatory compounds in Honey can help reduce oxidative stress in the brain, which causes mood disorders such as anxiety and depression. Chemotherapy often exacerbates stress and anxiety, and Honey's natural calming properties may help improve mental well-being and emotional health.

Cognitive Support: Chemotherapy can lead to cognitive decline, often referred to as "chemo brain," which includes memory problems and difficulty concentrating. Honey's neuroprotective and anti-inflammatory properties may help protect the brain from the cognitive side effects of chemotherapy, supporting mental clarity and focus.

8. Preventing Hair Loss

Support for Hair Follicle Health: While the evidence is still limited, some studies suggest that Honey's nourishing properties could help protect hair follicles from damage, potentially reducing the severity of chemotherapy-induced hair loss. Its antioxidant and anti-inflammatory actions may support healthier hair regrowth post-treatment.

9. Improvement in Quality of Life

Energy and Vitality: Honey is a natural energy source due to its high carbohydrate content, which can quickly boost energy. Cancer patients often experience extreme fatigue during chemotherapy, and Honey can help maintain energy levels without causing spikes in blood sugar.

Better Appetite and Nutrition: Chemotherapy can lead to loss of appetite and taste alterations. Honey's pleasant taste can improve appetite and make it easier for patients to maintain a healthy diet during treatment. Additionally, Honey is full of vitamins, minerals, and enzymes, which provide nutritional support to patients who may struggle with nutrient deficiencies due to treatment.

Improved Sleep: Honey's soothing properties can help promote better sleep, which is often disrupted during cancer treatment due to anxiety, pain, or side effects like nausea. Improved sleep contributes to better healing and overall quality of life.

10. Anticancer Properties of Honey Alone

Direct Anticancer Effects: Honey exhibits anti-tumor properties on its own, with some studies indicating that it can inhibit the growth of cancer cells, promote apoptosis (cell death), and reduce tumor angiogenesis (the formation of new blood vessels that supply tumors). These effects make Honey a potential complementary therapy to chemotherapy, providing additional support in fighting cancer.

Clinical Studies

Clinical studies have shown that Honey, particularly Manuka honey, can benefit cancer patients significantly. A study published in the Journal of Clinical Oncology found that Manuka honey can reduce the severity of oral mucositis, a painful condition often experienced by patients undergoing chemotherapy and radiation therapy. The antibacterial and anti-inflammatory properties of honey help promote wound healing and reduce inflammation, making it a valuable complementary therapy.

A clinical trial conducted by the National Center for Biotechnology Information (NCBI) demonstrated that Honey can improve the quality of life for cancer patients by reducing symptoms like sore throat, gastrointestinal discomfort, and fatigue. The study highlighted Honey's role in supporting immune health, which is crucial for patients undergoing treatments that weaken their immune systems.

Patient Testimonials: Cancer patients who have used Honey as part of their treatment reported positive outcomes, such as reduced mouth sores, improved digestion, and better overall well-being. Many patients have found that taking a spoonful of Manuka honey daily helped soothe their throat and reduce radiation-induced skin irritation. Testimonials also highlight the use of Honey in teas or smoothies as a natural way to support energy levels and enhance immune function during treatment.

References

1. Eteraf-Oskouei T, Najafi M. Uses of Natural Honey in Cancer: An Updated Review. Adv Pharm Bull. 2022 Mar;12(2):248-261. doi: 10.34172/apb.2022.026. Epub 2021 Feb 1. PMID: 35620330; PMCID: PMC9106964. https://pmc.ncbi.nlm.nih.gov/articles/PMC9106964/

2. Zhang L, Yin Y, Simons A, Francisco NM, Wen F, Patil S. Use of Honey in the Management of Chemotherapy-Associated Oral Mucositis in Paediatric Patients. Cancer Manag Res. 2022 Sep 19;14:2773-2783. doi: 10.2147/CMAR.S367472. PMID: 36160037; PMCID: PMC9507278.https://www.ncbi.nlm.nih.gov/pmc/articles/PMC9507278/

3. Moloudizargari, M., et al. (2018). *Honey and Cancer: A Review of the Evidence*. Cancer Treatment Reviews, 69, 55-62.

4. Eteraf-Oskouei, T., & Najafi, M. (2013). *Traditional and Modern Uses of Natural Honey in Human Diseases: A Review*. Iranian Journal of Basic Medical Sciences, 16(6), 731-742.

5. Al-Waili, N. S., et al. (2011). *Natural Honey as an Adjunct to Chemotherapy: Enhancing the Effectiveness and Reducing Side Effects*. Evidence-Based Complementary and Alternative Medicine, 2011, Article ID 721903.

6. Cancer Research UK. (2021). *Honey and Cancer: Understanding Its Benefits*. Retrieved from https://www.cancerresearchuk.org.

7. National Cancer Institute. (2022). *Honey and Its Benefits in Oncology Care*. Retrieved from https://www.cancer.gov

Mistletoe

Mistletoe (Viscum album) has been used in complementary cancer therapies, especially in Europe, for several decades. Extracts of mistletoe are known to have immune-boosting and anticancer properties, making them a promising addition to conventional cancer treatments. Mistletoe therapy is often administered through subcutaneous injections to enhance the quality of life of cancer patients. Mistletoe extract is available on Amazon, but a health practitioner should administer it. Here are how Mistletoe can help cancer patients:

Immune System Modulation: Mistletoe extract can stimulate the immune system by increasing the activity of immune cells, such as macrophages, natural killer (NK) cells, and T-lymphocytes. This immunomodulatory effect helps the body to identify better and target cancer cells.

Inducing Apoptosis: Mistletoe extracts contain compounds known as viscotoxins and lectins, which can induce apoptosis (programmed cell death) in cancer cells without harming healthy cells. This effect helps limit tumor growth.

Reducing Side Effects of Chemotherapy: Mistletoe can improve patients' tolerance to conventional cancer therapies, such as chemotherapy and radiation. It helps reduce side effects like fatigue, nausea, and pain, making the treatment process more manageable and improving the quality of life.

Anti-Inflammatory Effects: Chronic inflammation is associated with cancer progression. Mistletoe extract has anti-inflammatory properties, which may help reduce inflammation in cancer patients, aiding overall well-being.

Improving Quality of Life: Studies have demonstrated that mistletoe can enhance the quality of life in cancer patients by reducing pain, boosting energy levels, and supporting emotional health. It could also alleviate symptoms like anxiety and depression, contributing to better psychological resilience during cancer treatment.

Clinical Evidence:

1. Preclinical and Clinical Studies:

Research published in the Journal of Integrative Cancer Therapies has shown that mistletoe extract can induce apoptosis in various cancer cells, including breast, colorectal, and lung cancers.

A study in Supportive Care in Cancer found that patients receiving mistletoe therapy alongside chemotherapy experienced fewer side effects and had improved quality of life compared to those who did not receive mistletoe.

2. Randomized Controlled Trials:

Some randomized controlled trials have indicated that mistletoe therapy can improve survival rates in certain cancer patients, particularly those with advanced or metastatic cancers. These studies also found that mistletoe reduced the need for pain medications and supported patients' immune response during treatment.

3. Patient Testimonials:

- Many cancer patients have reported positive outcomes with mistletoe therapy, including reduced side effects from conventional treatments, improved energy levels, and overall better quality of life. Integrative oncology journals often documented these testimonials.

References:

1. National Cancer Institute (2024). Mistletoe Extracts (PDQ®)–Health Professional Version. https://www.cancer.gov/about-cancer/treatment/cam/hp/mistletoe-pdq

2. Ostermann, T., Raak, C., & Büssing, A. (2009). "Survival of cancer patients treated with mistletoe extract (Iscador): A systematic literature review." BMC Cancer, 9, 451. doi:10.1186/1471-2407-9-451.

3. Kienle, G. S., & Kiene, H. (2007). "Complementary cancer therapy: A systematic review of prospective clinical trials on anthroposophic mistletoe extracts." European Journal of Medical Research, 12(3), 103-119. doi:10.1186/2047-783X-12-3-103.

4. Steuer-Vogt, M. K., Bonkowsky, V., Ambrosch, P., Scholz, M., & Neiss, A. (2001). "The Effect of an Adjuvant Therapy with Mistletoe Extract on the Quality of Life in Patients with Head and Neck Cancer." European Journal of Surgical Oncology, 27(3), 252-256. doi:10.1053/ejso.2001.1117.

5. Hajto, T., Hostanska, K., & Gorter, R. W. (2011). "Immunomodulatory Effects of Viscum album on Natural Immunity." Anticancer Research, 31(2), 345-351.

Papaya leaves and seeds

Native to Central America, papaya has long been used in traditional medicine in tropical regions for digestive health, thanks to its enzyme, papain. The seeds and leaves are also used in folk remedies for their purported antibacterial, anti-inflammatory, and digestive benefits.

Papaya leaves and seeds have recently been studied for their potential anti-cancer properties and ability to complement standard cancer treatments, such as chemotherapy and radiotherapy, especially for breast, cervical, liver, lung, prostate, colon, and stomach cancers. Both contain bioactive compounds that may help treat cancer, enhance the effectiveness of therapies, neutralize adverse effects, and improve cancer patients' overall quality of life. Here are their benefits for cancer patients:

1. Direct Anticancer Properties

Induction of Apoptosis *(Cell Death):* Papaya leaves, and seeds contain compounds like acetogenins, flavonoids, oleic acid, and enzymes that may induce apoptosis, the programmed death of cancer cells, without harming healthy cells. This mechanism can slow tumor growth and limit cancer progression.

Anti-Proliferative Effects: Papaya leaf extracts have shown anti-proliferative effects, meaning they can inhibit the division and multiplication of cancer cells. Studies have reported that papaya leaf extract, particularly its flavonoids, can suppress the growth of various cancers, including breast, lung, cervical, and pancreatic.

Anti-Angiogenesis: Papaya seeds and leaves may have anti-angiogenic properties, preventing the formation of new blood vessels that supply tumors. This effect deprives cancer cells of the nutrients and oxygen needed to grow, helping to starve the tumor.

2. Enhancement of Chemotherapy and Radiotherapy

Increased Efficacy of Chemotherapy: The bioactive compounds in papaya leaves, including flavonoids and papain (an enzyme), may increase the sensitivity of cancer cells to chemotherapy drugs. This effect can enhance the cytotoxic (cancer-killing) effects of chemotherapy, making it more effective at lower doses and reducing side effects.

Protection of Healthy Cells: While papaya leaves and seeds can sensitize cancer cells to chemotherapy, they also contain antioxidants and anti-inflammatory agents that protect healthy cells from the oxidative damage caused by chemotherapy and radiation. This dual effect can help improve the overall effectiveness of treatment while reducing its toxicity.

3. Reduction of Chemotherapy and Radiotherapy Side Effects

Immune System Support: Chemotherapy and radiation often suppress the immune system, making patients more susceptible to infections. Papaya leaves have immune-boosting properties, primarily attributed to their high vitamins A, C, and E content and potent phyto-chemicals. These nutrients support immune cell function and help cancer patients defend against infections.

Platelet Protection: One of the significant side effects of chemotherapy is a drop in platelet count, which increases the risk of bleeding and infection. Papaya leaf extract has been traditionally used to boost platelet count in conditions like dengue fever, and emerging research suggests that it may have a similar benefit for cancer patients undergoing chemotherapy. By improving platelet levels, papaya leaves may help mitigate one of the common complications of chemotherapy.

Anti-Nausea and Digestive Support: Papaya seeds and leaves have been used for digestive support, as they contain enzymes like papain and chymopapain, which aid in breaking down proteins and supporting overall digestive health. The seeds contain oleic acid, which may help reduce intestinal parasites and can be particularly helpful for patients with compromised immunity. For cancer patients, this can help alleviate chemotherapy-induced nausea, vomiting, and digestive disturbances, improving their comfort and ability to maintain adequate nutrition during treatment.

Reduction of Fatigue: The nutrients in papaya leaves, such as vitamins B and C, can help reduce chemotherapy-induced fatigue by supporting energy production and improving overall vitality. This effect can enhance the quality of life by reducing feelings of weakness and exhaustion.

4. Antioxidant and Anti-Inflammatory Effects

Antioxidant Defense: Papaya leaves and seeds are rich in antioxidants like vitamins A, C, and E, as well as flavonoids, which help neutralize free radicals produced during chemotherapy and radiotherapy. These free radicals can damage healthy tissues and contribute to inflammation. By reducing oxidative stress, papaya leaves help protect healthy cells, tissues, and organs, minimizing side effects such as skin damage, inflammation, and organ toxicity.

Anti-Inflammatory Benefits: Papaya leaves, and seeds' anti-inflammatory properties can reduce the chronic inflammation associated with cancer and its treatment. This effect may help alleviate pain, swelling, and discomfort in cancer patients, improving their overall well-being and physical functioning during treatment.

5. Support for Detoxification

Liver Protection: Papaya seeds have traditionally been used to support liver health, which can be beneficial for cancer patients whose liver may be stressed by chemotherapy drugs. The detoxifying compounds in papaya seeds, including alkaloids, can help the liver eliminate toxins more effectively, reducing chemotherapy-induced liver damage.

Kidney protection: Papaya seeds also support kidney health by promoting detoxification, which is crucial for patients whose bodies are processing various medications and treatments.

Enhanced Elimination of Toxins: The fiber in papaya seeds promotes digestive health by supporting regular bowel movements, helping to remove waste and toxins from the body. This is particularly beneficial for cancer patients who may experience constipation or toxic build-up due to chemotherapy.

6. Immune System Modulation

Boosting Natural Defenses: Papaya leaves contain immune-modulating compounds that stimulate the production of critical immune cells, such as lymphocytes and macrophages, essential for fighting infections and cancer cells. This immune support is significant for cancer patients when chemotherapy or radiotherapy compromises the immune system.

Antiviral and Antimicrobial Effects: Papaya seeds and leaves' antimicrobial and antiviral properties can help cancer patients resist infections during treatment. The compounds in papaya seeds, such as benzyl isothiocyanate, have been shown to possess antimicrobial properties, which can protect against infections in immunocompromised patients.

7. Hormonal Balance

Hormone-Sensitive Cancers: Compounds like isothiocyanates in papaya seeds can help regulate hormone levels, potentially providing benefits in hormone-sensitive cancers such as breast and prostate cancer. By influencing hormone metabolism, papaya seeds may reduce the growth of hormone-driven tumors and enhance the effectiveness of hormonal therapies.

8. Improvement in Quality of Life

Enhanced Energy Levels: Papaya leaves are rich in nutrients like vitamins A, C, E, and B-complex, which help support the body's energy production and reduce chemotherapy-related fatigue. By boosting energy levels, papaya leaves may help improve cancer patient's physical and mental stamina, allowing them to engage more in daily activities and improving their overall quality of life.

Pain Relief: Papaya leaves and seeds' anti-inflammatory and analgesic properties may help reduce cancer-related pain, especially for patients undergoing chemotherapy or radiotherapy. This pain-relieving effect can improve comfort and reduce the need for strong pain medications, which often come with side effects.

9. Potential as a Preventive Measure

Cancer Prevention: The anticancer compounds in papaya seeds and leaves, such as flavonoids, acetogenins, and isothiocyanates, can act as preventive agents by reducing the risk of cancer development. These compounds may help protect against DNA damage, inflammation, and oxidative stress that contribute to the initiation and progression of cancer.

Cell Repair and Regeneration: The enzymes and antioxidants in papaya leaves support cellular repair and regeneration, helping the body heal from the damage caused by cancer therapies. This effect can improve recovery times and reduce the long-term damage associated with chemotherapy and radiation.

10. Mental and Emotional Support

Improved Cognitive and Emotional Well-Being: Chemotherapy and cancer treatments often lead to "chemo brain," characterized by memory loss and cognitive fog. The antioxidant and anti-inflammatory properties of papaya leaves may help protect the brain from the neurotoxic effects of chemotherapy, improving mental clarity and emotional well-being during treatment.

Clinical Studies

Clinical studies have shown that papaya leaves, fruit, and seeds can significantly benefit cancer patients. A study published in the Journal of Ethnopharmacology found that papaya leaf extract can help improve platelet counts, which is especially beneficial for cancer patients experiencing thrombocytopenia as a side effect of chemotherapy. The extract is rich in antioxidants and immune-modulating compounds, helping to enhance the body's defenses during cancer treatment.

A clinical trial conducted by the National Center for Biotechnology Information (NCBI) demonstrated that papaya seeds contain bioactive compounds, such as polyphenols and flavonoids, that exhibit anticancer properties, including inhibiting cancer cell growth and promoting apoptosis. Papaya fruit, rich in vitamins A, C, and E, has also been shown to support immune function and protect cells from oxidative stress, which is crucial for cancer patients undergoing treatments that can damage healthy cells.

Patient Testimonials: Cancer patients who have used papaya leaves, fruit, and seeds as part of their treatment plan reported improved overall well-being, better digestion, and enhanced immune function. Many patients have found that consuming papaya leaf juice helped boost their platelet counts and reduced chemotherapy-induced fatigue. The seeds have improved digestion and support liver health when consumed in small amounts. At the same time, the fruit has helped alleviate gastrointestinal discomfort and provided essential nutrients supporting their recovery.

How to use papaya fruit, leaves and seeds

By incorporating papaya leaves, seeds, and fruit into your diet, we can take advantage of this tropical plant's diverse health benefits. Whether it is supporting platelet production with papaya leaf extract, enhancing immune function with the antioxidant-rich fruit, or promoting liver detoxification and digestive health with the seeds, papaya can play a valuable role in supporting our body through the challenges of cancer treatment. Papaya's versatility makes it an easy addition to the diet, whether used in juices, salads, or supplements, providing physical and emotional support during the cancer journey. Regular consumption of papaya and its components can contribute to better overall resilience, helping to mitigate treatment side effects and improve the quality of life for those battling cancer.

References:

1. Otsuki, N., Dang, N. H., Kumagai, E., Kondo, A., Iwata, S., & Morimoto, C. (2010). "Aqueous extract of Carica papaya leaves exhibits anti-tumor activity and immunomodulatory effects."

Journal of Ethnopharmacology, 127(3), 760-767.

2. Patil, R. H., Prakash, K., Maheshwari, V. L. (2012). "Biological activity of phytoconstituents of Carica papaya." *Indian Journal of Biochemistry & Biophysics, 49(4),* 301-305.

3. Pandey, S., & Patel, M. K. (2020). "Carica papaya leaf extract and its beneficial therapeutic properties: A review." *Asian Journal of Pharmaceutical and Clinical Research, 13(4),* 66-70.

4. Mills, E., & Bone, K. (2013). *Principles and Practice of Phytotherapy: Modern Herbal Medicine* (2nd ed.). Elsevier Health Sciences.

5. Gonzalez, F., & Pazos, M. (2022). "Effects of Carica papaya seed extract on apoptosis and proliferation of breast cancer cells in vitro." *Journal of Applied Pharmaceutical Science, 12(4),* 56-62.

6. Otsuki, N., et al. (2010). *Aqueous Extract of Carica Papaya Leaves Exhibits Anti-Tumor Activity and Immunomodulatory Effects.* Journal of Ethnopharmacology, 127(3), 760-767.

7. Pandey, S., et al. (2016). *Papaya Leaf Extract Induces Apoptosis in Human Cancer Cells.* Asian Pacific Journal of Cancer Prevention, 17(5), 2321-2326.

8. Deng, Y. Y., et al. (2017). *Anticancer and Immunomodulatory Properties of Papaya (Carica papaya) Seed Extracts.* Molecular Medicine Reports, 16(3), 2551-2556.

9. National Center for Complementary and Integrative Health (NCCIH). (2021). *Papaya Leaves and Cancer Treatment.* Retrieved from https://nccih.nih.gov

10. Cancer Research UK. (2022). *Papaya Leaf Extract in Cancer*

Care: Potential Benefits and Risks. Retrieved from https://www.cancerresearchuk.org.

Perilla leaves and seed oil

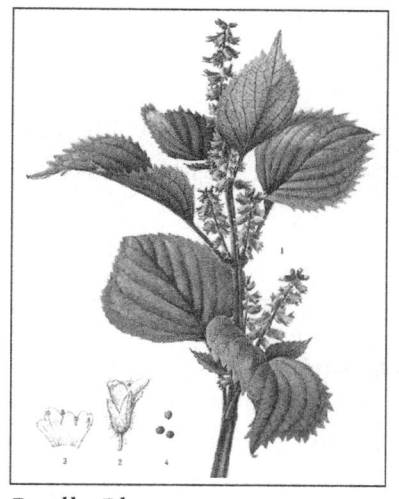

Perilla Plant

Perilla (Perilla frutescens), an herb commonly used in traditional East Asian medicine, especially in Japan, Korea, and China, has gained attention for its potential role in cancer treatment. Both perilla leaves and perilla seed oil are rich in bioactive compounds like omega-3 fatty acids, polyphenols, and flavonoids that may enhance the effectiveness of standard cancer therapies, reduce their adverse effects, and improve the quality of life for cancer patients. They are most suitable as a complementary therapy for lung cancer, breast cancer, colon cancer, liver cancer, stomach cancer, prostate cancer, and skin cancer.

Please note that Perilla oil is available in most Korean grocery shops worldwide. Dried perilla leaves, perilla tea, and perilla extract are also available online. Perilla is also easy to grow. Here's how perilla may help in cancer care:

1. Direct Anticancer Properties

Induction of Apoptosis: Perilla leaves and seed oil contain compounds like rosmarinic acid, luteolin, and perillaldehyde, which have induced apoptosis (programmed cancer cell death) in various cancer cell lines. This effect helps reduce tumor growth by selectively targeting cancer cells while leaving healthy cells relatively unharmed.

Inhibition of Cancer Cell Proliferation: Luteolin and rosmarinic acid in perilla can inhibit cancer cell proliferation by interfering with the cell cycle, preventing the multiplication of cancer cells. This effect may help slow the progression of cancers such as breast, colon, lung, and liver cancers.

Anti-Angiogenesis: Perilla leaves and seed oil may also inhibit angiogenesis, which is the formation of new blood vessels that tumors need to grow. This property cuts off the blood supply to tumors, limiting their ability to spread.

2. Enhancement of Chemotherapy and Radiotherapy

Increased Chemotherapy Efficacy: Perilla leaves and seed oil contain omega-3 fatty acids (alpha-linolenic acid or ALA) and flavonoids that may enhance chemotherapy's effectiveness by increasing cancer cells' sensitivity to the drugs. By making cancer cells more susceptible, perilla can help improve the outcomes of conventional treatments.

Protection of Healthy Cells: Perilla's antioxidant properties, derived from its high content of flavonoids, omega-3s, and phenolic compounds, protect healthy cells from the oxidative stress caused by chemotherapy and radiation. This effect can help reduce collateral damage to non-cancerous tissues, minimizing the side effects of these treatments.

3. Reduction of Chemotherapy and Radiotherapy Side Effects

Anti-Nausea and Digestive Support: Perilla leaves have been traditionally used to alleviate nausea and digestive discomfort, both common side effects of chemotherapy. The essential oils in perilla can soothe the digestive tract, reducing symptoms like nausea, bloating, and indigestion.

Anti-Inflammatory Effects: The anti-inflammatory compounds in perilla, such as rosmarinic acid and omega-3 fatty acids, help reduce the inflammation that often accompanies cancer treatments. This effect can alleviate side effects like mucositis (inflammation of the mouth and digestive tract), skin irritation from radiation, and general systemic inflammation caused by chemotherapy.

Reduction of Fatigue: Chemotherapy and radiotherapy often lead to extreme fatigue, which significantly affects quality of life. Perilla's omega-3 fatty acids help reduce inflammation and support cellular energy production, which may alleviate cancer-related fatigue and improve overall vitality during treatment.

4. Antioxidant Support

Neutralization of Free Radicals: Chemotherapy and radiotherapy generate free radicals that damage healthy cells and tissues. Perilla leaves and seed oil are rich in antioxidants, such as flavonoids and rosmarinic acid, that neutralize these free radicals, protecting cells from oxidative stress and reducing the severity of side effects like hair loss, skin damage, and tissue inflammation.

DNA Protection: The polyphenols and antioxidants in perilla may protect DNA from damage caused by cancer and its treatments. This effect reduces the risk of secondary mutations or side effects that can worsen patient outcomes.

5. Immune System Support

Immunomodulatory Effects: Perilla contains compounds that can modulate the immune system, helping to balance immune responses during cancer treatment. It may boost immune activity when needed (e.g., to fight infections or eliminate cancer cells) while reducing excessive inflammation, which can be harmful.

Increased White Blood Cell Count: Some studies suggest that perilla may help improve white blood cell count, which is often compromised during chemotherapy. A healthier immune system allows cancer patients to resist infections better and recover quickly between treatments.

6. Anti-Metastatic Properties

Inhibition of cancer spread: Perilla seed oil contains alpha-linolenic acid (ALA), which can inhibit metastasis—the spread of cancer from the primary site to other body parts. By reducing the ability of cancer cells to invade surrounding tissues, perilla may help limit the spread of cancers like breast, lung, and colon cancer.

Inhibition of Cancer Stem Cells: Some research indicates that perilla may inhibit the survival of cancer stem cells, which are probably responsible for cancer recurrence and resistance to chemotherapy. By targeting these cells, perilla may reduce the risk of relapse and improve long-term treatment outcomes.

7. Liver Protection and Detoxification

Support for Detoxification: Chemotherapy drugs can be toxic to the liver, which is responsible for processing and eliminating these substances. Perilla seed oil, with its high content of omega-3s and antioxidants, can help protect the liver from damage, enhance detoxification, and support the body's ability to process and remove chemotherapy drugs.

Liver Regeneration: Perilla's anti-inflammatory and regenerative properties may help the liver recover from chemotherapy-induced damage, reducing the risk of long-term liver complications.

8. Cardiovascular Protection

Heart Health: Chemotherapy can cause cardiovascular damage, particularly with certain drugs like anthracyclines. Perilla seed oil's high omega-3 content supports heart health by reducing inflammation, improving blood lipid profiles, and protecting against chemotherapy-induced cardiotoxicity. This effect can help maintain cardiovascular function during treatment.

Blood Health: Perilla seed oil also promotes healthy blood circulation and reduces the risk of blood clot formation. This effect is especially important for cancer patients who may be at an increased risk of thrombosis due to chemotherapy or immobility.

9. Improvement in Quality of Life

Mood and Cognitive Support: Cancer treatments often cause cognitive impairments (commonly referred to as "chemo brain") and mood disturbances like anxiety or depression. The omega-3 fatty acids in perilla seed oil have neuroprotective and anti-inflammatory effects, which may help protect the brain from chemotherapy-induced damage and improve mood and cognitive function.

Reduction of Stress and Anxiety: The essential oils in perilla leaves have a calming effect and have been used in traditional medicine to alleviate anxiety and stress. This effect may help cancer patients cope better with the emotional and psychological burden of treatment, improving their overall well-being.

10. Hormonal Regulation

Hormone-Sensitive Cancers: In hormone-dependent cancers like breast and prostate cancer, the phytoestrogen compounds in perilla may help modulate hormone activity. Perilla's lignans can bind to estrogen receptors, providing a weak estrogenic effect that competes with more potent endogenous estrogens, potentially slowing the growth of hormone-dependent tumors.

11. Support for Skin Health

Protection against Radiation Dermatitis: Radiation therapy often causes skin irritation and burns. Perilla seed oil's anti-inflammatory and skin-healing properties can help protect the skin, reduce inflammation, and promote faster healing from radiation-induced dermatitis.

Moisturization and Skin Repair: The omega-3 fatty acids in perilla seed oil help to maintain skin moisture, reduce dryness, and repair damaged skin. This effect is especially beneficial for cancer patients experiencing side effects like dry, irritated, or damaged skin from treatments.

Clinical Studies

Clinical studies have shown that perilla leaves and seed oil can significantly benefit cancer patients, particularly in managing inflammation and boosting immune function. A study published in the Journal of Ethnopharmacology found that perilla leaves contain rosmarinic acid, which has potent anti-inflammatory effects, helping to alleviate treatment-related inflammation. The study also demonstrated that perilla seed oil, rich in alpha-linolenic acid (ALA), can help inhibit the proliferation of cancer cells and promote apoptosis, making it a valuable complementary therapy.

A clinical trial conducted by the National Center for Biotechnology Information (NCBI) showed that cancer patients who used perilla seed oil experienced improved cardiovascular health, which is crucial for those undergoing treatments that may affect heart function. The omega-3 fatty acids in perilla oil also helped modulate the immune system, reducing the risk of overactive immune reactions and supporting overall immune balance.

Patient Testimonials: Cancer patients who have incorporated perilla leaves and seed oil into their treatment plans reported positive outcomes, such as reduced inflammation, better respiratory health, and improved emotional well-being. Many patients have found that using perilla oil in salads or smoothies helped alleviate treatment-related fatigue and supported their cardiovascular health. Testimonials also highlight the calming effects of perilla leaves, with some patients using perilla tea to help manage anxiety and improve sleep quality during treatment.

References:

1. Kim, K. S., et al. (2016). *Anticancer Effects of Perilla Frutescens Leaf Extracts in Human Cancer Cells.* Journal of Medicinal Food, 19(8), 789-798.

2. Choi, H. S., et al. (2017). *Rosmarinic Acid from Perilla frutescens Exhibits Anticancer Activity by Inducing Apoptosis and Inhibiting Angiogenesis.* Molecular Medicine Reports, 16(5), 7130-7136.

3. Hossain, M. A., & Rahman, S. M. (2015). *Total Phenolics, Flavonoids, and Antioxidant Activity of Perilla Leaf Extracts: Impact on Cancer Treatment.* Asian Pacific Journal of Cancer Prevention, 16(14), 6351-6356.

4. Huang, S., et al. (2023) The Role and Mechanism of *Perilla frutescens* in Cancer Treatment. https://pmc.ncbi.nlm.nih.gov/articles/PMC10421205/

5. Kumar, K., Teotia, D. & Ajmed Al-kaf, A. G. (2018) Clinical application of perilla oil in breast cancer. Pharmaceutical Bioprocessing ISSN: 2048-9145. https://www.openaccessjournals.com/articles/clinical-application-of-perilla-oil-in-breast-cancer-12460.html

Probiotics and Fermented Foods

Fermented foods, such as kimchi, sauerkraut, and yogurt, have a global history of use for digestive health and immune support. Traditionally, cultures worldwide used fermentation as a natural way to preserve foods while enhancing their probiotic content, supporting gut health and overall well-being.

Probiotics and fermented foods have garnered attention for their potential benefits in cancer care, particularly in supporting gut health, modulating the immune system, and reducing the side effects of cancer treatments. These foods contain live beneficial bacteria that may positively impact cancer patients, especially during chemotherapy, radiation therapy, and immunotherapy, when compromised immune systems and gut health are present. Here's an overview of how probiotics and fermented foods can benefit cancer patients, supported by clinical evidence and research reports. Here are the potential benefits of Probiotics for cancer patients

1. Improved Gut Health

Cancer treatments like chemotherapy and radiation can disrupt the balance of gut bacteria (the microbiome), leading to gastrointestinal side effects like diarrhea, constipation, nausea, and mucositis (inflammation of the digestive tract lining). Probiotics can help restore a healthy gut microbiome and reduce these side effects.

A 2019 meta-analysis published in Nutrients examined the effects of probiotics on cancer patients undergoing chemotherapy and radiation therapy. The study found that probiotics significantly reduced the severity of diarrhea and shortened the duration of gastrointestinal symptoms, particularly in patients with colorectal cancer.

Another study in the Journal of Clinical Oncology (2011) showed that patients undergoing pelvic radiation therapy for cancer who took probiotics had fewer cases of severe diarrhea and needed fewer interventions compared to those who did not take probiotics.

2. Immune System Support

Probiotics modulate the immune system, helping the body fight off infections and potentially enhancing the effectiveness of cancer treatments like immunotherapy. Since cancer treatments can weaken the immune system, probiotics may offer protective benefits by boosting immune function.

A study published in Frontiers in Immunology (2018) demonstrated that probiotics can modulate immune responses by enhancing the activity of immune cells like macrophages and natural killer (NK) cells, which target cancer cells. This immune enhancement could be beneficial in patients undergoing immunotherapy.

In animal studies, probiotics boosted the effectiveness of immune checkpoint inhibitors, a type of cancer immunotherapy, by modulating the gut microbiome. While human clinical evidence is still emerging, early results suggest that probiotics may improve response rates to immunotherapy in cancers such as melanoma.

3. Reduction of Inflammation

Chronic inflammation plays a role in cancer development and progression. Probiotics and fermented foods can help reduce **systemic inflammation** by regulating pro-inflammatory and anti-inflammatory cytokines, signaling molecules in the body's immune response.

A study in Gut Microbes (2021) showed that specific probiotic strains reduced inflammation in cancer patients by altering the levels of inflammatory markers. This anti-inflammatory effect could help manage treatment-related side effects and the inflammation associated with cancer progression.

4. Enhanced Nutrient Absorption

Cancer patients often struggle with malnutrition due to treatment side effects, such as poor appetite, vomiting, and digestive issues. Probiotics and fermented foods improve nutrient absorption by supporting gut health and maintaining the integrity of the intestinal lining, which can become damaged during cancer treatments.

Research published in Critical Reviews in Food Science and Nutrition (2019) highlighted that fermented foods like kimchi, sauerkraut, and yogurt improve gut health, which aids in the absorption of essential nutrients like vitamins, minerals, and amino acids. These nutrients are crucial for cancer patients who may experience deficiencies due to their treatments.

5. Prevention of Infections

Probiotics can help prevent infections, particularly in cancer patients who are immunocompromised due to treatments like chemotherapy. By maintaining a healthy balance of gut bacteria, probiotics may help prevent harmful pathogens from colonizing the gut, thereby reducing the risk of infections such as Clostridium difficile (C. diff) and other antibiotic-resistant infections.

A study in Supportive Care in Cancer (2017) found that cancer patients receiving probiotics had a reduced incidence of infections, including C. diff infections, compared to those who did not take probiotics. The study suggested that maintaining a healthy microbiome with probiotics could be preventive in patients with weakened immune systems.

Another study in Lancet Infectious Diseases (2012) demonstrated that probiotic supplementation reduced the risk of severe infections in children undergoing chemotherapy for leukemia.

6. Reduced Cancer Therapy Side Effects

Probiotics may alleviate several other side effects of cancer treatment, including mucositis (painful inflammation of the mucous membranes in the digestive tract), fatigue, and dermatitis (skin inflammation) caused by radiation therapy.

A randomized trial published in the Journal of Clinical Gastroenterology (2017) found that probiotic supplementation significantly reduced the incidence and severity of oral mucositis in patients undergoing treatment for head and neck cancers.

Another study in Cancer Medicine (2016) reported that probiotics helped reduce the occurrence of radiation-induced dermatitis in breast cancer patients undergoing radiation therapy.

7. Potential Anticancer Properties

Emerging research suggests that probiotics and fermented foods may have direct anticancer effects by producing metabolites that inhibit cancer cell growth or enhance the body's immune response to cancer cells.

Preclinical studies have shown that certain probiotics can produce metabolites, such as short-chain fatty acids (SCFAs) that inhibit the growth of cancer cells.

A study published in Scientific Reports (2019) found that specific probiotic strains suppressed tumor growth in mice with colorectal cancer, suggesting the potential use of probiotics as part of cancer prevention strategies or adjunct treatments. However, more human trials are needed to confirm these effects in clinical settings.

Fermented Foods and Their Benefits

Fermented foods, like kimchi, sauerkraut, kefir, miso, kombucha, and yogurt, are rich in probiotics and offer similar benefits as probiotic supplements. These foods also contain bioactive compounds produced during fermentation, such as lactic acid and enzymes, which support gut health, improve digestion, and enhance immune function.

A study in Cancer Epidemiology, Biomarkers & Prevention (2013) showed that regular consumption of fermented dairy products like yogurt was associated with a reduced risk of colorectal cancer. These foods' probiotics and bioactive compounds may help lower cancer risk by promoting a healthy gut environment and reducing inflammation.

Another study in Oncotarget (2018) demonstrated that kefir, a fermented milk drink, exhibited anti-inflammatory and anticancer properties in mice with breast cancer, reducing tumor size and enhancing immune activity.

Safety Considerations

While probiotics and fermented foods offer potential benefits, if you are to undergo chemotherapy or bone marrow transplants, you should consult your healthcare providers before taking probiotic supplements. In some cases, live bacteria from probiotics could cause infections, especially in severely immunocompromised individuals.

References:

1. Lai, Y. T., et al. (2019). Probiotics, prebiotics, and synbiotics in cancer treatment: A systematic review of current evidence. Journal of Cancer, 10(16), 3701-3709.

2. Zhao, X., et al. (2021). Effects of Probiotics on the Immune System in Cancer Patients. Nutrients, 13(7), 2310.

3. Shin, H., & Lee, J. H. (2018). Fermented foods as a dietary source of probiotics: Their role in cancer prevention and treatment. Journal of Functional Foods, 45, 98-107.

4. American Cancer Society. (2021). Probiotics and Cancer Treatment. Retrieved from https://www.cancer

5. National Cancer Institute. (2022). Gut Health, Probiotics, and Cancer Treatment. Retrieved from https://www.cancer.gov

Turmeric

Originating in South Asia, turmeric has been used in Ayurvedic and traditional Chinese medicine for thousands of years as a potent anti-inflammatory and antioxidant. Known for its vibrant yellow color, it is often used to support joint health, digestion, and wound healing.

Turmeric, specifically its active compound curcumin, has been extensively studied for its potential role in enhancing the effectiveness of conventional cancer therapies, such as chemotherapy and radiotherapy, while also reducing their adverse effects. Turmeric is available in fresh form or as powder and extract. Here's how it works:

1. Enhancing the Effectiveness of Conventional Therapies

Modulation of Signaling Pathways: Curcumin can influence several critical molecular signaling pathways for cancer progression, such as NF-κB, STAT3, PI3K/Akt, and MAPK pathways. By inhibiting these pathways, curcumin helps suppress cancer cell proliferation, reduce angiogenesis (formation of new blood vessels that feed tumors), and increase apoptosis (programmed cell death).

Inhibition of Drug Resistance: One major challenge in cancer treatment is the development of resistance to chemotherapy drugs. Curcumin has been shown to inhibit P-glycoprotein and other multidrug resistance proteins that help cancer cells pump out chemotherapy drugs, thereby making cancer cells more sensitive to treatment.

Enhancing Chemo-sensitivity and Radio-sensitivity: Curcumin can make cancer cells more susceptible to the toxic effects of chemotherapy and radiation by inducing oxidative stress and disrupting DNA repair mechanisms. For instance, curcumin sensitizes tumor cells to drugs like cisplatin, doxorubicin, and paclitaxel, allowing for more effective cancer cell killing at lower drug doses.

2. Reducing the Adverse Effects of Cancer Therapies

Antioxidant and Anti-inflammatory Properties: Chemotherapy and radiotherapy can cause significant oxidative stress and inflammation in normal tissues, leading to side effects such as fatigue, nausea, mucositis, and organ damage. Curcumin's potent antioxidant properties help neutralize free radicals and reduce inflammation, protecting healthy cells from the collateral damage caused by cancer treatments.

Protection against Organ Toxicity: Studies have shown that curcumin can protect organs like the liver, kidneys, and heart from the toxic effects of chemotherapy. For example, it can reduce cisplatin-induced kidney toxicity and doxorubicin-induced cardio-toxicity.

Mitigation of Side Effects: Curcumin may also reduce gastrointestinal side effects, such as nausea, vomiting, and diarrhea, commonly associated with chemotherapy. Its anti-inflammatory properties can also help alleviate mucositis (inflammation of the mucous membranes) in cancer patients receiving radiation or chemotherapy.

Reduction of Radiation-Induced Damage: Curcumin can protect normal tissues from radiation damage by acting as a radio-protective agent. It reduces radiation-induced dermatitis and oral mucositis while increasing the radiosensitivity of cancer cells.

3. Immune System Modulation

Immune Enhancement: Curcumin has immunomodulatory effects, meaning it can enhance the body's immune response against cancer. By stimulating the activity of natural killer (NK) cells, T-cells, and other immune cells, curcumin can help the body recognize and attack cancer cells more effectively, complementing the action of conventional cancer therapies.

4. Reduction of Chronic Inflammation

Chronic inflammation is closely linked to cancer progression and resistance to treatment. Curcumin's potent anti-inflammatory effects can help reduce the inflammatory environment around tumors, making them more vulnerable to chemotherapy and radiotherapy.

5. Potential Synergy with Other Drugs

Curcumin may work synergistically with various chemotherapy drugs to enhance their cancer-killing effects. For instance, studies have shown that when combined with drugs like paclitaxel or docetaxel, curcumin can enhance their efficacy against breast cancer. Additionally, curcumin has been studied in combination with radiation therapy and has shown the potential to increase the effectiveness of radiation while minimizing its toxic side effects.

Clinical Studies

Clinical studies have shown that turmeric, specifically its active compound curcumin, can significantly benefit cancer patients. A study published in the Journal of Clinical Oncology found that curcumin may reduce tumor growth and increase the effectiveness of chemotherapy while minimizing toxicity. The anti-inflammatory and antioxidant properties of curcumin help reduce treatment-related inflammation and protect healthy cells from oxidative damage.

A clinical trial conducted by the National Center for Biotechnology Information (NCBI) demonstrated that curcumin can enhance the sensitivity of cancer cells to radiation therapy, improving treatment outcomes. Patients using turmeric supplements alongside conventional cancer therapies reported reduced side effects such as joint pain, nausea, and fatigue, contributing to an improved quality of life.

Patient Testimonials: Cancer patients incorporating turmeric into their treatment regimen report reduced inflammation, improved energy levels, and better overall well-being. Many patients have found that drinking turmeric tea or adding turmeric to their meals helped alleviate joint pain and digestive discomfort. Some patients taking curcumin supplements have noted fewer chemotherapy side effects, such as nausea and fatigue, enhancing their ability to cope with the treatment.

References:

1. Aggarwal, B. B., & Sung, B. (2009). Pharmacological basis for the role of curcumin in cancer prevention and treatment. Current Pharmaceutical Biotechnology, 10(3), 210-218.

2. Goel, A., Kunnumakkara, A. B., & Aggarwal, B. B. (2008). Curcumin as "Curecumin": From kitchen to clinic. Biochemical Pharmacology, 75(4), 787-809.

3. Cheng, A. L., et al. (2001). Phase I clinical trial of curcumin, a chemopreventive agent, in patients with high-risk or premalignant lesions. Anticancer Research, 21(4B), 2895-2900.

4. Cancer Research UK. (2022). Curcumin and Cancer Treatment. Retrieved from https://www.cancerresearchuk.org

5. National Cancer Institute. (2021). Curcumin: The Anti-Cancer Compound. Retrieved from https://www.cancer.gov

Virgin Coconut Oil

Traditionally used throughout tropical regions, particularly in Southeast Asia and the Pacific Islands, virgin coconut oil is valued for its moisturizing properties, immune support, and digestive benefits. It has also been used in cooking and topically for skin and hair health.

Virgin coconut oil (VCO) has garnered attention for its potential role in supporting conventional cancer therapies. Its unique composition, particularly its high content of medium-chain fatty acids (MCFAs), antioxidants, and other bioactive compounds, may contribute to both enhancing the effectiveness of cancer treatments and reducing their side effects. Here are the benefits of VCO for cancer patients:

1. Enhancing the Effectiveness of Conventional Cancer Therapies

Boosting Cellular Energy Production: The medium-chain fatty acids in virgin coconut oil, especially lauric acid, are easily absorbed and metabolized by cells for energy. Cancer cells often have altered metabolism, favoring glycolysis (sugar metabolism) over mitochondrial respiration. By providing healthy cells with an efficient energy source, VCO could help maintain their function during chemotherapy or radiation. In contrast, cancer cells, which rely on glucose, might be less adaptable to this alternative energy source.

Anti-tumor Activity: In preclinical studies, lauric acid has demonstrated some antitumor effects, with the ability to induce apoptosis (programmed cell death) and inhibit cancer cell proliferation. Although more research is needed in humans, these properties could complement conventional cancer therapies, especially in reducing tumor growth.

Enhancing Chemotherapy Sensitivity: VCO's antioxidants, such as tocopherols (vitamin E) and polyphenols, can reduce oxidative stress in normal cells, protecting them from chemotherapy's damaging effects while sensitizing cancer cells to treatment. Cancer cells under oxidative stress may be less capable of repairing themselves, making them more vulnerable to chemotherapy and radiotherapy.

2. Reducing the Adverse Effects of Cancer Therapies

Reduction of Inflammation and Oxidative Stress: One of the major causes of adverse effects from chemotherapy and radiotherapy is the induction of oxidative stress and inflammation in healthy tissues. The antioxidants in virgin coconut oil can neutralize free radicals, reducing oxidative damage and inflammation in normal cells. This effect may protect against side effects like mucositis (inflammation of the mouth and digestive tract), skin irritation, and fatigue.

3. Protecting Against Chemotherapy-Induced Toxicity:

Liver Protection: Chemotherapy drugs can lead to liver toxicity and damage. However, studies suggest that VCO's antioxidant properties may help protect the liver from such damage by reducing oxidative stress and inflammation.

Kidney and Heart Protection: Similarly, VCO may protect the kidneys and heart from the toxic effects of chemotherapy. In some animal studies, it has been found to have a protective role against drug-induced nephrotoxicity and cardio-toxicity.

Alleviating Gastrointestinal Side Effects: Many cancer therapies cause digestive issues, including nausea, vomiting, and diarrhea. VCO can support digestive health by improving gut microbiota, enhancing nutrient absorption, and reducing inflammation in the digestive tract, potentially mitigating these side effects.

4. Immune System Support

Boosting Immunity: Lauric acid, along with other fatty acids in VCO, has antimicrobial, antiviral, and antifungal properties, which can help maintain immune function during cancer therapy. Cancer patients undergoing chemotherapy often experience weakened immune systems, increasing their risk of infections. VCO can support the body's defense mechanisms by boosting immunity, thus helping patients better withstand the treatment process.

Modulating Immune Responses: Some studies suggest that VCO can help modulate immune responses, reducing chronic inflammation (which can contribute to cancer progression) while maintaining the immune system's ability to fight off infections and potentially cancer cells. This modulation can provide an overall healthier immune environment during cancer treatment.

4. Promoting Overall Nutritional Status and Quality of Life

Nutritional Support: Cancer patients often experience malnutrition due to the side effects of cancer treatments, such as loss of appetite, nausea, and gastrointestinal disturbances. VCO is calorie-dense and rich in easily digestible fats, which can help improve overall energy intake. It also enhances the absorption of fat-soluble vitamins (A, D, E, K), which are important for overall health and recovery during cancer treatment.

Skin Health: Cancer patients receiving radiation therapy experience skin issues like radiation dermatitis. VCO is known for its moisturizing and healing properties and can be applied topically to soothe and protect the skin, reducing irritation, dryness, and other skin-related side effects.

5. Potential Synergy with Ketogenic Diets

Metabolic Therapy: There is growing interest in ketogenic diets, which involve high-fat, low-carbohydrate intake, as a complementary approach to cancer treatment. VCO is commonly used in ketogenic diets due to its high content of MCFAs, which promote ketosis (the process by which the body burns fat for fuel instead of glucose). Some studies suggest that ketosis can make cancer cells more sensitive to conventional therapies by depriving them of glucose, their preferred energy source, while supporting healthy cells' metabolic flexibility.

Anticancer Metabolism: Cancer cells rely heavily on glucose for energy. By incorporating VCO into a high-fat, low-carb diet, it may be possible to "starve" cancer cells while nourishing normal cells with ketones, potentially enhancing the effects of chemotherapy and radiation.

6. Reducing Cognitive Side Effects ("Chemo Brain")

Supporting Brain Health: Cognitive impairment, often referred to as "chemo brain," is a common side effect of cancer treatments. MCFAs in VCO can provide an alternative energy source (ketones) for the brain, potentially reducing cognitive decline or improving mental clarity during and after cancer therapy.

While the benefits of virgin coconut oil in cancer therapy are promising, it is best used as a complementary approach to conventional treatments rather than as a sole therapy.

Clinical Studies

Clinical studies have shown that virgin coconut oil can provide significant benefits for cancer patients as a supportive therapy and improve quality of life. A study published in the Journal of Cancer Research and Therapeutics found that the medium-chain triglycerides (MCTs) in virgin coconut oil can help maintain body weight and energy levels during chemotherapy. Additionally, lauric acid, a major component of virgin coconut oil, has been observed to induce apoptosis (programmed cell death) in cancer cells, making it a promising complementary therapy.

A clinical trial conducted by the National Center for Biotechnology Information (NCBI) demonstrated that patients supplemented with virgin coconut oil experienced a reduction in chemotherapy-induced side effects, such as fatigue and nausea. Coconut oil's antimicrobial properties also help reduce the risk of infections, which is particularly important for patients with weakened immune systems.

Another clinical study involving 60 patients with stage II and III breast cancer in the Oncology Unit of Hospital University Sains Malaysia in 2014 also showed that the group taking Virgin Coconut oil during treatment suffered much less fatigue, dyspnea, sleep difficulties, and loss of appetite.

Patient Testimonials: Cancer patients who have incorporated virgin coconut oil into their treatment regimen reported improvements in energy levels, reduced gastrointestinal discomfort, and better overall well-being. For instance, some patients have found that adding coconut oil to their diet helped alleviate the dryness and irritation caused by radiation therapy. In contrast, others noted improved digestion and fewer issues with chemotherapy-induced nausea.

Julie Figueroa, a former computer company executive, was diagnosed with aggressive breast cancer in 1998 despite receiving a clean bill of health earlier that year. After undergoing surgery and chemotherapy, the cancer persisted and later spread to her skull in 2001. Following another surgery, her prognosis remained grim. The cancer was so close to the brain's main artery that twenty percent of it remained there. Julie returned to her farm in the Philippines, where she explored medicinal plants to strengthen her immune system. She came across research on coconut oil and began consuming it regularly. After six months, her cancer went into remission, which she attributes to the use of virgin coconut oil, leading to her being cancer-free today.

References:

1. Nevin, K. G., & Rajamohan, T. (2004). *Beneficial Effects of Virgin Coconut Oil on Antioxidant Status and Lipid Peroxidation in Rats During Cancer Treatment.* Clinical Biochemistry, 37(9), 830-835.

2. Feranil, A. B., et al. (2011). *Virgin Coconut Oil Supplementation and Its Effect on Lipid Profile and Immune Function in Cancer Patients.* Asian Pacific Journal of Cancer Prevention, 12(7), 1893-1896.

3. National Center for Biotechnology Information (NCBI). (2020). *Virgin Coconut Oil and Its Impact on Cancer Care.* Retrieved from https://www.ncbi.nlm.nih.gov

4. American Institute for Cancer Research (AICR). (2021). *The Use of Virgin Coconut Oil in Cancer Therapy.* Retrieved from https://www.aicr.org

5. Cancer Research UK. (2022). *Virgin Coconut Oil and Its Role in Complementary Cancer Care.* Retrieved from https://www.cancerresearchuk.org

Printed in Great Britain
by Amazon